Praise for
AIDS AND THE DOCTORS OF DEATH

"Who should read AIDS AND THE DOCTORS OF DEATH?
Every man and woman on this planet!"
— Wildfire Magazine

"A provocative book that should cause more than a few waves
of doubt in the troubled seas of AIDS research."
— East-West Magazine

"Riveting, I couldn't put it down!"
— Health and Healing Magazine

"When Cantwell implicates agencies like the National Cancer
Institute in a shadowy antigay conspiracy ... his argument de-
serves thoughtful consideration."
— Wilson Library Bulletin

"A well-written, entertaining book for those who love myster-
ies and conspiracies ... not to mention ... scientific matters."
— Update Magazine

"Though the accusations are startling, the book is unlike many
'alternative medicine' books in that the author has scientific
credentials ... reference sources ... respected journals ... to
back up his theories."
— The Kirkwood News

Distributed by:
Baker & Taylor, Inland, New Leaf, and Bookpeople.

Also by
Alan Cantwell Jr., M.D.

AIDS: THE MYSTERY & THE SOLUTION
THE CANCER MICROBE
QUEER BLOOD

AIDS AND THE
DOCTORS OF DEATH

AIDS

AND THE DOCTORS OF

DEATH

AN INQUIRY INTO THE
ORIGIN OF THE AIDS EPIDEMIC

ALAN CANTWELL JR., M.D.

FOREWORD BY JON RAPPOPORT

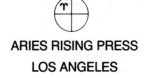

ARIES RISING PRESS
LOS ANGELES

Cover design by Ron Anderegg © 1987

Printed in the United States of America

Library of Congress Cataloging-in-Publication Data

Cantwell, Alan, 1934-
    AIDS and the Doctors of Death: An inquiry into the
    origin of the AIDS epidemic / Alan Cantwell Jr:
    foreword by Jon Rappoport
    p. cm
    Includes bibliographies and indexes
    1.AIDS (Disease)—Etiology
    AIDS (Disease)—Epidemiology
    1. Title

RC607.A26C35 1988 616.9'792-dc19 87-37355

ISBN 0-917211-25-1 (softcover)
ISBN 0-917211-00-6 (hardcover)

10 9 8 7 6 5

"When your body and your ego and your dreams are gone, you will know that you will last forever. Perhaps you think this is accomplished through death, but nothing is accomplished through death, because death is nothing. Everything is accomplished through life, and life is of the mind and in the mind. The body neither lives nor dies, because it cannot contain you who are life."

—A Course in Miracles

CONTENTS

ACKNOWLEDGMENTS

This book is an outgrowth of a meeting in the summer of 1986 that became one of the most signficant events in my life. I am indebted to my longtime friend and mentor, Virginia Livingston-Wheeler, M.D., and her husband, Owen Wheeler, M.D., for inviting me to that special event where I first heard a serious discussion of the theory of AIDS as a biowarfare experiment.

Judy Dowd, Linda Yokoyama, and Jeff Elzer of the Kaiser Foundation Hospital Medical Library in Los Angeles, helped immeasurably in securing much of the medical reference material used in this project.

During the intense year of writing the manuscript, many friends offered valuable bits of AIDS-related information from newspapers, magazines, and other sources that have become incorporated into this book. Among these friends are: Armand Auger, M.D., Orin Borsten, Edward George Garren, Verne Haddon, Barry Lynes, Evelyn Nadel, Howard Quande, Frank A. Sinatra, Millard Tipp, and Jack True.

I am honored that Jon Rappoport consented to write the Foreword. Jon's seminal reports on the origin of AIDS have appeared in numerous magazines and newspapers, and are among the most provocative and controversial reports ever published on the AIDS epidemic.

A special thanks goes to Ron Anderegg for his artistic talents in designing the book jacket, and for his support of this project.

My editor, Professor Suzanne Henig, provided invaluable literary expertise and penetrative analyses of certain portions of the manuscript that resulted in alterations that greatly improved the final quality of this book.

Finally, I extend my deepest gratitude to Robert Strecker, M.D. In the year that I have known him he has affected my life in awesome ways because of his unique concept of the origin of AIDS. He has become my friend and my teacher, and has opened my mind to a wealth of scientific material that has completely changed my own views of the AIDS situation.

In many ways, this book is Strecker's.

I appreciate this opportunity to share some controversial views of AIDS with others, in the hope that new thought and renewed ideals will help conquer the most dastardly disease ever unleashed on the planet.

Foreword

If you nose around and ask a lot of questions for a few months, you begin to get a new slant on this disease called AIDS. You begin to wonder seriously whether all possible explanations of the disease are getting a fair shake.

Like any other institution, the AIDS-research establishment is run by a small group of people; its representatives dispense information to the press about the latest breakthroughs, possible cures, etc.

Science writers of the working press take their cues from these reps, and the assumption is that these writers are getting the latest and greatest news and there isn't any other news.

That, of course, cuts across the grain of the inquiring reporter who likes to investigate a little. Well, most of us start off by assuming that people in charge of anything are of good will. We believe the Authorities are trying to do their best, always. We think our leaders are less

1

interested in politics than truth.

Then something happens; a scandal, a mess, a ridiculous embarrassment. The curtain is lifted on a piece of disgusting news and we change our minds.

Researching AIDS makes one wonder.

Why are people at the National Institutes of Health (NIH) only interested in one theory of the disease when there are four or five kicking around out there that deserve funding and study?

Is the point to cure the disease—or to keep the research in the hands of a few men who can command huge amounts of Congressional funding?

Clearly, in order to assure lots of research dollars, scientists have to keep a proper face on their efforts. They can't admit weakness, uncertainty. They have to forge ahead with their HIV (AIDS) virus and their questionable plans for a vaccine, a magic bullet that will wipe the AIDS problem off the face of the earth.

Ask any ten working scientists about the chances of AIDS originating by accident in a lab...and ten will scoff at you. The look you get will say, "Why, how perfectly crude of you to suggest such a thing. How absurd. Only an uneducated non-Ph.D. without a credential to his name would suggest such tripe."

Fact is, in 1987 the collective Lab around the world consists of thousands of rooms and tens of thousands of experiments. Fact is, this collective Lab is a jungle of its own, an immense reservoir of viruses, lost and found, contaminating cell-lines and experiments more than once in a while.

It's a perfectly sensible doubt to have: could AIDS have escaped from a lab? Worldwide, laboratory accidents and safety violations occur frequently. When a new disease pops

2

up like AIDS, the Lab is one of the first places one ought to look.

Scientists, of course, don't want to open the door to the possibility that they could have contributed to illness and death.

In the last months that I've been researching AIDS and writing articles on it, nothing has convinced me that our so-called top scientists have a handle on the disease. And privately, a few university scientists have admitted as much to me.

Read Michael Gold's book, *A Conspiracy of Cells* (1986). See how, when a few scientists are confronted with their own sloppiness, their own botched experiments, their own wasted time and money—see how they mainly refuse to admit the truth, watch how they try to lie and discredit the source of the accusations, watch how they act like a bunch of low-life hustlers whose shell-game has been burned. Watch what happens to the vaunted idea of Truth.

Read this book by Alan Cantwell. He doesn't swallow the party-line about AIDS as the word from the good gods.

He's inclined to doubt. That's what I like about him. He doesn't accept the premise that our guardians of science are always speaking sooth. At the same time, *he* admits he doesn't have all the answers either.

Cantwell doesn't try to pull rank on people by telling them he's a *doctor*. He doesn't burn the academic incense and invoke his degrees and look down at you from some non-existent ladder.

Before this thing is over, we may well find that AIDS has something to do with microbe-messing...the kind that goes on in labs, in the manufacture of vaccines, in the shooting up of animals with all sorts of germs that come from the species of other animals...

Cantwell knows something about all of this. He isn't a guy who defends the scientific throne always and forever. He'll tell you things you ought to think about. Listen to him.

—Jon Rappoport
Los Angeles, August 1987

(Jon Rappoport is a free-lance reporter. He has written for *Stern*, *In These Times*, *Village Voice*, *New York Native*, *LA Weekly*, *Sports International*, and other newspapers in the U.S. and Europe. Currently, he has been writing articles on the origin of AIDS.)

CHAPTER ONE

The Myth of "Gay" Cancer

From the very beginning of the epidemic of AIDS (acquired immune deficiency syndrome), I was never satisfied with the theories which attempted to explain how the disease started in America and elsewhere in the world. Part of the reason for my dissatisfaction stemmed from what I had learned about cancer and so-called "gay cancer," long before anyone had ever heard of AIDS.

In 1981, Kaposi's sarcoma became widely known as "gay cancer" because it was often found in homosexual men with AIDS. The distinctive, purple-red skin tumors of Kaposi's quickly became one of the major signs of this new and deadly disease which had a strange affinity for young white gay men.

Few people understood the paradox that linked Kaposi's sarcoma to AIDS, and the jumbling of scientific facts which connected "gay" cancer to this "new" disease called AIDS.

In actuality, Kaposi's sarcoma was a century-old form of cancer which was discovered in 1872 in Vienna, Austria, by the famous dermatologist Moriz Kaposi. Before the AIDS epidemic, "classic" Kaposi's was a rare form of cancer, found primarily in people whose familial

origins stemmed from eastern Europe and the Mediter-
ranean. Several decades ago, Kaposi's sarcoma was
discovered to be a very common cancer in central
Africa.

Most doctors tend to have explicit trust in the
scientific pronouncements of high-ranking "authority
figures" in medical science. It is rare to find physicians
who challenge established thinking, and it is profession-
ally very risky to do so. However, my unusual experiences as a physician-dermatologist and cancer researcher
made me highly skeptical of certain aspects of AIDS
"science." As a consequence, I often found the "official"
AIDS dogma at odds with my own scientific beliefs.

For over three decades I had studied certain kinds of
cancer and other immunologic diseases in a very special
way. During those years, I proved to my own satisfaction
that easily visible "cancer bacteria" were involved in
causing these diseases. I wrote over thirty published
scientific papers which presented this important information to medical doctors and the scientific world.

I first learned about the "cancer microbe" from
Doctor Virginia Livingston-Wheeler, whom I met in the
early 1960s. After becoming acquainted with her vast
research and scientific publications in the field of cancer
microbiology, I began my own personal study of cancer
bacteria as possible cancer-causing agents.

Since my initial meeting with Doctor Virginia, I have
had the honor of meeting other physicians and scientists
who have also devoted their lives to uncovering the
secrets of the microbe of cancer. Among this group are
Eleanor Alexander-Jackson of New York City, Irene

Diller of Philadelphia, Florence Seibert of St. Petersburg, Georges Mazet of Cannes, and others.

I also became aware of little-known cancer scientists like Royal Rife who invented a powerful microscope which demonstrated these cancer germs as far back as the 1930s. I was amazed to learn of the cancer studies of Wilhelm Reich who discovered "bions" — particles of energy that are clearly related to cancer bacteria. Over the years, I have learned about other obscure scientists who also believed that cancer bacteria were the cause of cancer. I wrote about some of these pioneer cancer microbiologists in my book, *AIDS: The Mystery & The Solution*, (1984).

Scientists like Rife and Reich suffered greatly and paid dearly for challenging the medical establishment with their revolutionary discoveries and treatment methods for cancer.

Rife was driven to alcoholism by the government's relentless efforts to prosecute him for discovering a possible cancer cure. Reich died in Federal prison while serving a jail sentence imposed on him by a government court when he refused to cooperate with the Federal Drug Administration (FDA). BEFORE INCARCERATING HIM IN 1957, FDA OFFICIALS AXED REICH'S INSTRUMENTS AND BURNED HIS BOOKS AND JOURNALS. THE DESTRUCTION OF WILHELM REICH'S LABORATORY BY THE U.S GOVERNMENT WAS LIKE A SCENE OUT OF NAZI GERMANY, BUT IT HAPPENED IN AMERICA.

Harsh governmental action against intransigent and "unorthodox" physicians and scientists serves to maintain the "status quo" of orthodox American medical practice. Challenges to official governmental authority in matters of cancer research and treatment are simply not tolerated.

It is clear to anyone who has studied the matter that the medical "establishment," along with its intimate connections to the pharmaceutical industry and federal agencies such as the FDA, is opposed to any "breakthrough" or "cure" for serious chronic diseases like cancer and AIDS. According to various official sources, the direct treatment costs for cancer now total 60 billion dollars per year. The average medical and hospitalization costs for each AIDS patients is $150,000. It is not difficult to understand why a breakthrough for cancer and AIDS could jeopardize the multi-billion dollar, government-sanctioned cancer and AIDS industry in America.

Before AIDS became well-known in 1981, I had spent several years studying "classic" Kaposi's sarcoma skin tumors in three elderly men who were patients in my dermatology clinic practice. As part of a research project, I carefully searched the specially-stained microscopic sections of their cancer tumors for the presence of cancer bacteria.

With the assistance of Dan Kelso, a microbiologist, we cultured the Kaposi's skin cancer tumors for bacteria. And with Jerry Lawson, a pathologist, we studied an autopsied case of an elderly man who died of Kaposi's in 1973. Prior to AIDS, it was very uncommon for a patient to die of this form of cancer. However, this particular man suffered for two years with increasing tumors of Kaposi's, as well as opportunistic infections, before dying of this rare disease.

Before AIDS began, my microbiologic research into the cause of "classic" Kaposi's sarcoma convinced me of three important things.

First, I discovered that *bacteria* could be seen microscopically in Kaposi's tumors when the tissue was stained in a special way.

Second, the microbes that I observed in the tumors were similar to *cancer bacteria* which had been previously discovered in other forms of cancer by other scientists.

And third, the microbes I saw in Kaposi's cancer tumors could be grown and cultured in a bacteriology laboratory.

Shortly after the epidemic began, I studied the "gay" Kaposi's sarcoma tumors which appeared on the skin of homosexuals with AIDS. When their tissue sections were colored with an "acid-fast" stain and examined microscopically, I recognized the same bacteria that I had seen in the skin tumors of my three, non-gay men with "classic" Kaposi's.

When homosexual men died of AIDS at our institution, I examined their autopsy tissue. To my surprise, *I found widespread evidence of cancer bacteria in the AIDS-damaged tissue.*

During the years 1981-1986, the results of this research were published in scientific journals. All 7 medical reports contained pictures of cancer bacteria that were observed and cultured from "classic" and "gay" Kaposi's sarcoma, and from AIDS tissue.

Although these remarkable discoveries were published

in reputable, peer-reviewed journals, no AIDS "expert" has ever commented on them publicly. Despite the seriousness of the new epidemic and the millions of dollars spent on AIDS research, the discoveries of cancer bacteria in AIDS, Kaposi's sarcoma, and cancer remain ignored. Undoubtedly, the main reason that these bacteria remain ignored is that physicians have been carefully taught that bacteria are not the cause of cancer and AIDS.

When the epidemic first broke out, government scientists were convinced that AIDS was a *new disease* caused by a *new infectious agent,* most probably a *virus.* Scientists did not bother to look for viruses in the regular light-microscope because viruses are too small in size to be seen with that instrument. Researchers did not look for bacteria in Kaposi's sarcoma because medical scientists do not believe that cancer bacteria exist in any form of cancer, including Kaposi's.

The AIDS experts were all hunting for a "new" virus in AIDS. I kept wondering how a brand-new virus could be causing a century-old form of cancer. It didn't make any sense.

In 1984, when the AIDS virus was "officially" discovered, scientists insisted the new virus was the "sole" cause of AIDS. *However, the new virus was not the cause of Kaposi's sarcoma.* I couldn't understand how the AIDS virus could be the "sole" cause of AIDS if the virus didn't cause Kaposi's sarcoma! I was also amazed at the rapidity with which Kaposi's became widely known as "gay" cancer. How could an old form of cancer suddenly become "gay?"

The AIDS experts quickly assured the public that AIDS was not cancer (even though it could lead to cancer). But my research had convinced me that *AIDS was cancer*! I suspected the reason the scientists didn't want to tell the public that AIDS was cancer is because doctors had always insisted that cancer was not contagious or infectious. However, the public was informed that this new kind of "gay" cancer was catching! Somehow, homosexuals had proved the impossible.

After the AIDS virus was discovered, and after a blood test was designed to test for AIDS virus antibodies, it was undeniable that the "new" virus was involved in the new disease AIDS. More and more medical reports attested to its lethal effects. Even though I finally accepted the reality of the new, immunosuppressive and cancer-causing AIDS virus, I knew there was much more to AIDS than merely the AIDS virus.

The end results of AIDS and cancer were the same. I had studied autopsies of people who died of cancer, and I studied autopsies of people who died of AIDS. There was no substantial difference between them.

I could see cancer bacteria in patients who died of cancer. And I could see these same bacteria in gays who died of AIDS. It was incredible that no one else seemed interested in studying these microbes that I could see so clearly.

After the discovery of the AIDS virus in 1984, the virologists began to theorize that the new virus originated in central Africa in African green monkeys. Their story was that the monkey AIDS virus "jumped species" and entered the black African population. From there, the deadly virus supposedly made its way to Haiti. After spreading through heterosexual contacts in Africa and Haiti, the virus suddenly entered the gay male population of Manhattan.

Scientists theorized that traveling gay New Yorkers had picked up the virus during anal intercourse with Haitian men. After acquiring the virus in Haiti, the gays brought it back to America. Once introduced into other promiscuous New York City gays, the virus than spread to hemophiliacs, drug addicts, and into the "general" population.

To my mind, much of AIDS "science" was tinged with madness. In spite of the "brilliant" discovery of the AIDS virus, and the assertions that scientists had learned "a great deal" about the disease, in actuality they knew little, if anything, about AIDS. The mounting death toll of the "invariably fatal disease" (over 20,000 deaths by 1987) was proof of that.

With my knowledge of cancer microbes, I remained highly skeptical of the theories the AIDS experts so eagerly supplied to the media, theories that were quickly parroted into fact by physicians and science writers alike.

The sensational AIDS stories were a journalist's dream. Reporters wrote of a new and deadly sexually-transmitted agent that lurked in the sinful world of the homosexual; a world of semen and sodomy, drugs and promiscuity, and life in the fast lane.

As a physician and cancer researcher, I knew there was no such thing as "gay cancer," and no such thing as a virus that targeted only gay men. As a dermatologist, I had studied many different kinds of infectious and contagious microbes that caused venereal disease. Before AIDS, there had never been an infectious agent that attacked only one small segment of society, such as young white homosexual men in Manhattan.

It was impossible for such a thing to happen. And yet it did happen.

There were many unanswered questions about AIDS that were deeply disturbing to me.

WHY DID AIDS BEGIN EXCLUSIVELY AS A GAY DISEASE?

WHY WOULDN'T THE AIDS EXPERTS ADMIT THEY WERE DEALING WITH AN EPIDEMIC OF CANCER?

AND WHY WOULDN'T SCIENTISTS PAY ATTENTION TO MICROBES IN AIDS AND KAPOSI'S?

In time, I was to discover frightening answers to these questions.

References:

Cantwell AR Jr: Bacteriologic investigation and histologic investigation of variably acid-fast bacteria in three cases of cutaneous Kaposi's sarcoma. Growth 45: 79-89, 1981.

Cantwell AR Jr, Lawson JW: Necroscopic findings of pleomorphic, variably acid-fast bacteria in a fatal case of Kaposi's sarcoma. J Dermatol Surg Oncol 7: 923-930, 1981.

Cantwell AR Jr: Variably acid-fast bacteria in vivo in a case of reactive hyperplasia occurring in a young male homosexual. Growth 46; 331-336, 1982.

Cantwell AR Jr: Necroscopic findings of variably acid-fast bacteria in a fatal case of acquired immunodeficiency syndrome and Kaposi's sarcoma. Growth 47: 129-134, 1983.

Cantwell AR Jr: Kaposi's sarcoma and variably acid-fast bacteria in vivo in two homosexual men. Cutis 32: 58-64, 1983.

Cantwell AR Jr, Rowe L: African "eosinophilic bodies" in vivo in two American men with Kaposi's sarcoma and AIDS. J Dermatol Surg Oncol 11: 408-412, 1985.

Cantwell AR Jr: Mycobacterium avium-intracellulare infection and immunoblastic sarcoma in a fatal case of AIDS. Growth 50: 32-40, 1986.

Cantwell A Jr: *AIDS: The Mystery and the Solution,*

Aries Rising Press, Los Angeles, 1984.

Wuerthele-Caspe (Livingston) V, Alexander-Jackson E, Anderson JA, et al. Cultural properties and pathogenicity of certain microorganisms obtained from various proliferative and neoplastic diseases. Amer J Med Sci 220: 628-646, 1950.

Wuerthele-Caspe Livingston V, Livingston AM: Demonstration of Progenitor cryptocides in the blood of patients with collagen and neoplastic diseases. Trans NY Acad Sci 34(5): 433-453, 1972.

Wuerthele-Caspe Livingston V, Livingston AM: Some cultural, immunological, and biochemical properties of Progenitor cryptocides. Trans NY Acad Sci 36(6): 569-582, 1974.

Livingston VWC: *Cancer, A New Breakthrough,* Nash Publishing Corp, Los Angeles, 1972.

Alexander-Jackson, A: A specific type of microorganism isolated from animal and human cancer. Bacteriology of the organism. Growth 18: 37-51, 1954.

Seibert FB, Yeomans F, Baker JA, et al: Bacteria in tumors. Trans NY Acad Sci 34(6): 504-533, 1972.

Mazet G: Corynebacterium, tubercle bacillus, and cancer. Growth 38: 61-74, 1974.

Lynes B, Crane J: *The Cancer Cure That Worked (The Rife Report),* Marcus Books, Toronto, Canada, 1987.

Reich W: *The Cancer Biopathy,* Ferrar, Straus, and Giroux, New York, 1973.

Sharaf MR: *Fury On Earth. A Biography of Wilhelm Reich,* St. Martin's Press, New York, 1983.

Moss RW: *The Cancer Syndrome,* Grove Press Inc, New York, 1980.

CHAPTER TWO

The Meeting
with Strecker

By the spring of 1986, my curiosity about the *exclusive* origin of AIDS in the gay community became increasingly tinged with anger as I watched more and more friends, acquaintances, and patients die from this disease. Unbelievably, there was nothing anyone could do to save these men. The medical and scientific communities were powerless against the onslaught of the new virus.

In some ways, the beginning decimation of the gay community reminded me of the extermination of the Jews during the Nazi reign of terror. Although the enemy in AIDS was not human, it seemed to be capable of killing selectively. To be a Jew in Nazi Europe meant death; to be a gay man in New York, San Francisco, or Los Angeles now meant you had a fifty-fifty (or even greater) chance of dying of AIDS within a few years.

With the ever-expanding epidemic, many gays now live with fear, despair, and depression, with little hope for the future. Like the Jewish communities in Nazi Europe, the gay communities in America are slowly disappearing.

One night, my friend Gregg and I were bemoaning the deaths of so many people we knew who had died of

AIDS. After talking awhile, Gregg became greatly agitated. He surprised me by saying things I had never been told before. Lightly pounding his fist on the table, he raised his voice in anger.

"This whole AIDS thing is genocide. You must know they are trying to kill us all. They don't care how many of us die. Just look around. There are plenty of people who want to put us away in camps to die."

I couldn't believe he was serious. He continued on about the CIA, and how gay men were being used as guinea pigs, and how they gave the gays the AIDS virus.

Finally, I interrupted. "You don't just *give* somebody a virus. A virus like the AIDS virus would have to be injected. How the hell would someone go around injecting gays with the AIDS virus when it wasn't even discovered until five years *after* the epidemic started."

Gregg couldn't explain exactly how such a thing could have happened. However, he thought for a moment and said, "Well, you know there are VD clinics for gays. Somebody could have put AIDS in with the drugs they inject. It's not impossible, you know."

As a physician, I thought Gregg's ideas were ridiculous. It was preposterous talk. I was certain there was no way AIDS could have happened that way. We were both upset and changed the subject. Although it was disconcerting to hear Gregg's strange notions, I knew there were others who shared his belief that foul play was somehow connected with the AIDS epidemic stalking the gay community.

Months earlier, someone anonymously sent me a manuscript bizarrely titled *The AIDS Conspiracy — Corporate Murder.* There was no author's name on the manuscript. It was dated "Anno Domani, 1986."

The story gave me an uneasy feeling. It read: "AIDS has been definitely introduced into the United States. AIDS is a man-made disease. It did not evolve on its own nature. It has been scientifically engineered and developed for introduction into human populations. It is a variant of germ warfare. The gays, prostitutes, and drug addicts were initially marked for sacrifice so that the conspirators could accomplish their purposes in spreading the disease."

The manuscript was shocking and provocative. The author (or authors) accused big international interests "and their allies in the U.S. government, Big Oil, Big Banks, Major Chemical and Pharmaceutical Houses, the Medical and Dental Establishment, and the Intelligence Community," of deliberately introducing AIDS into America.

Despite the detailed presentation of these mind-boggling ideas, the idea of a deliberate "AIDS plot" was just too far-out for me. I simply could not believe that anyone or any group would be crazy enough to start an epidemic of AIDS.

Of course, I was prejudiced. My own research convinced me that AIDS was cancer. Nothing more, nothing less. The AIDS virus was undoubtedly real. It zeroed in on the white blood cells and eventually destroyed the immune system. But I was sure it was the cancer bacteria that killed people with AIDS. In my mind, AIDS was not a "new" disease. It was an "old" disease called cancer. The only difference was that it was now appearing in a highly aggressive, and sexually-transmitted way.

By the summer of 1986, I was in a mood to cool my preoccupation with the AIDS epidemic. The study of the disease and the writing of my AIDS book had consumed most of my spare time since 1981. I knew I had important contributions to make about the cause of AIDS, but very few people seemed interested in my ideas.

The AIDS experts had figured it all out, and they didn't want any conflicting theories which would cast doubt on their own. The science of AIDS had become a big business saturated with medical politics, and I have always hated medical politics with a passion.

I decided it was time to get away from AIDS, and to do something else with my life. But apparently this was not meant to be. Soon I would be meeting Strecker, and thinking about the epidemic in a way that I had never done before.

I remember distinctly the early morning phone call from Dr. Virginia Livingston-Wheeler that started it all in August 1986. At the age of 79, Virginia was a human dynamo, still working full-time at the medical clinic she founded in San Diego, and still proclaiming (to anyone who would listen) that the "cancer microbe" was the cause of cancer.

For forty years she had studied cancer bacteria. She showed them in every cancer tumor she investigated, as well as in the blood of cancer patients. She and her colleagues grew the cancer germs in her laboratory, and injected them into animals where they caused cancer. Over the past four decades, several dozen medical reports on her work were published in reputable journals, but still nothing came of it.

It was the same old story. Anytime a researcher without "official" grants or connections gets close to the cause or an effective treatment for cancer, they are ignored and/or censored by the medical establishment. If necessary, they are incarcerated by the federal authorities. Virginia has encountered all these experiences (except for the latter) as a result of her cancer research. Nevertheless, she continues to promote her idea of a "cancer microbe," and has devised a successful program for the prevention and treatment of cancer, which is outlined in her book, *The Conquest of Cancer*, (1984). She is a very gutsy lady.

Although she has highly respectable medical credentials, she is considered a "quack" by many physicians (and the American Cancer Society) because of her "unorthodox" cancer treatment methods (diet, megavitamins, and immuno-enhancing vaccines) as well as for her belief in a cancer "germ."

In my view, Dr. Virginia is an overlooked scientific genius, whose brilliant achievements in cancer microbiology will eventually pave the way for a cure for cancer and AIDS. For almost a quarter of a century she has been my friend and my mentor.

My own cancer and AIDS research was a natural outgrowth of her discoveries of a "cancer microbe" in cancer. My admiration for her scientific work is endless, and when Virginia speaks, I listen carefully.

After a brief hello, Virginia quickly got to the point.

"Alan, I have just heard the most dreadful thing. I've been in touch with a medical doctor in Los Angeles, and he says the whole AIDS virus thing was deliberately set and engineered."

She went on and on, rapidly talking about an AIDS conspiracy and a cover-up.

My mind was racing to keep up with her. What in God's name was she talking about? I couldn't believe she could be duped into such nonsense. She was sounding like my friend Gregg.

Finally, I interrupted. "Virginia, it sounds pretty far-out. Do you really think it's possible? I've heard that sort of thing before, but I never paid any attention to it."

Despite my objections, she continued.

"I want you to come down to San Diego this weekend to meet this doctor. His name is Robert Strecker. Some other doctors will be here too. You must come."

There was no use arguing with Virginia.

"OK, I'll be there."

After hanging up, I wondered what was going on. Virginia was no fool.

Why was this conspiracy thing popping up again-and-again in my life? Could there be anything to it?

I had to admit the conspiracy idea held a certain fascination for me. But so did James Bond, Sherlock Holmes, and the Hardy Boys. They were fantasies; AIDS was real.

Maybe this time I should just shut up and listen. After all, Virginia did say Strecker was a physician. I had never known a physician who believed that AIDS was "engineered." It was all rather exciting in a bizarre sort of way. Finally, I had to admit I was curious to hear what this M.D. from L.A. would say about AIDS.

As I headed down to San Diego with my closest

friend, Frank, I kept wondering what the day would bring. Sensing my increasing nervousness and fidgetiness as we neared the end of our trip, Frank finally said, "Relax! You haven't seen Virginia in ages. It should be an interesting meeting. And you know you've been dying to find out more about this AIDS conspiracy thing. Now's your chance."

My uneasiness settled a trifle once we found ourselves pleasantly chatting with an interesting group of people in the living room of Virginia and Owen Wheeler's spectacular hilltop home overlooking the ocean, and eagerly awaiting our mystery guest. Virginia said that Dr. Strecker had called to say he would be arriving a bit late. I found myself getting impatient. This meeting to discuss an AIDS conspiracy seemed so unreal.

Robert Strecker finally arrived, carrying two large cartons filled with hundreds of scientific papers on AIDS, cancer viruses, and genetic engineeering. He was powerfully built, and his energy filled the room. Strecker moved about the group quickly, giving each of us a vigorous handshake and a warm smile. There was something boyish about him, although he looked to be in his early forties.

He had an interesting medical background. He graduated from Vanderbilt University Medical School in 1974 with both an M.D degree and a Ph. D. in pharmacology. He studied internal medicine for four years at the University of Missouri, and followed that with two years of gastroenterology training and a three-year residency program in pathology at the University of Southern California. In short, he was a well-trained and a well-educated physician, hardly the sort to be discounted as a kook.

After the introductions and social amenities, Strecker quickly got down to business. He explained that he began his AIDS investigation two years previously when he and his brother, Ted, decided to look into the possibility of starting a health maintainance organization (HMO) group insurance plan. As a lawyer, Ted would research the legal problems, and Bob would try to figure out the health insurance cost per member.

The brothers soon found the issue of AIDS and AIDS-related illnesses to be a difficult and eventually insurmountable problem in terms of pre-planning future health care costs. This worrisome issue finally made them decide to abandon their health insurance business project.

But in the process of their AIDS research, they became convinced that the AIDS virus and the AIDS epidemic were not accidents of nature. On the contrary, their library research strongly suggested that the AIDS virus was deliberately unleashed as a "bioweapon attack" upon an unsuspecting public.

I was dumbfounded. I simply didn't know what to think. Never had I heard such bizarre ideas from a physician.

Perhaps sensing the group's disbelief, Strecker began to pass out copies of a report entitled "This is a Bio-Attack Alert." The manuscript was dated March 28, 1986, and was written by the Strecker brothers. The report contained detailed information on their theory, and provided documented evidence to show that the AIDS epidemic was biological warfare.

Months earlier, the Streckers had mailed "the Alert"

to over one hundred important government officials, warning them of the dangers of this biological warfare experiment. Copies were sent to all 50 state governors, as well as the President and Vice-President, all the Cabinet members, the head of the CIA and the FBI. According to Strecker, only three governors acknowledged the report, and promised to show it to their advisors. Strecker asked us to study the Bio-Attack report at our leisure.

Then Strecker carefully explained the unique molecular composition of the AIDS virus, emphasizing how it greatly resembles a virus in sheep called "visna virus."

In addition to having similarities to visna virus, the AIDS virus also has certain characteristics of a cattle retrovirus known as "bovine leukemia virus." According to Strecker's library research, the AIDS virus is so different in structure from any known virus that there is NO WAY it could have been formed by "mother nature."

He concluded that the AIDS virus must be a "man-made" and a "bioengineered" virus. The "new" AIDS virus was most probably created by splicing or mixing together two different viruses (like visna virus and bovine leukemia virus). When introduced into human beings, this totally new "recombined" AIDS virus was capable of producing a "new" disease.

Much of what Strecker was saying was way over my head, even though he was trying hard to make us understand. The highly technical scientific jargon of the virologists and immunologists is rarely understood by people outside the field. As a consequence, it requires a good deal of "faith" to believe in their scientific conclusions.

As Strecker expounded on the intricacies of the AIDS virus, I patiently awaited the opportunity to question him on his conspiracy theory. If there was a government plot against gay people, I wanted to know about it.

Finally I asked him the question that had brought me to San Diego on that fateful day.

"Apparently you believe that AIDS might have been deliberately set as some sort of biological warfare experiment. Tell me, how did gays get exposed to the AIDS virus?"

Strecker looked me straight in the eye, and without hesitating for a moment said, "It's very simple. They put it in."

I couldn't believe what I was hearing.

"What do you mean? They put it in? How?"

Strecker continued. "You remember the hepatitis B vaccine trials in New York City. It could have been done then."

I vaguely remembered the *experimental* vaccine trials which used gay men as volunteers back in the 1970s. A few years ago when physicians were urged to take the *commercial* hepatitis B vaccine, I requested it at the hospital where I work. I received a series of three injections with the vaccine.

I was sure the vaccine was perfectly safe. I certainly wouldn't have taken it if it were dangerous.

I protested to Strecker, "The vaccine is safe. I've taken it myself."

He responded, "Of course, the *commercial* hepatitis vaccine is safe. The AIDS virus was probably put into the *experimental* vaccine that was injected into gay volunteers. It was only the gays who got the virus. They wouldn't put it in an approved *commercial* vaccine for the general public!"

"That's ridiculous," I said. "If AIDS had been injected into gays in the hepatitis vaccine experiments, the epidemiologic experts would have traced it back to the original experiments. I remember reading somewhere that the gay men who were injected with the vaccine had the *same* incidence of AIDS as those who didn't get the vaccine. You know, the control group that got the placebo."

Unfazed by my comments, Strecker continued with his scenario. "What you don't understand is that the AIDS virus could have been given to *both* groups, the ones who got the vaccine and the ones who got the placebo. If that were the case, you wouldn't be able to detect any difference between the two groups."

The man seemed to have a lot of pat answers to some very complicated questions.

I found myself getting angry at his cock-sure attitude.

"Strecker, who would do such a crazy thing? And why?"

Sensing my anger, he said thoughtfully, "I don't know who did it. But there's no doubt in my mind that someone could have deliberately or accidentally sabotaged the vaccine trials in gays. I'm pretty sure that's how the AIDS virus was introduced into the gay community. There's no other logical explanation. And that's exactly what they wanted to do. It's in the medical literature, and it's in my Bioattack Report. Read it, and think about it for a while."

The group was mesmerized at the depth of Strecker's knowledge. He had obviously done his homework, and his contention that the AIDS epidemic was deliberately engineered was profoundly disturbing to us all.

After several heated hours of discussion followed by an early dinner, the group was weary. Before departing for the return trip to Los Angeles, we all agreed to meet again in the near future. Strecker promised to photocopy some of his important papers for us, and we would each try to read as much material as we could to prepare for the next meeting.

During the long trip back from San Diego with Frank, I was wired. I couldn't stop thinking about Strecker. Was he on to something, or was he some crazy, paranoid guy? I had met several truly nutty physicians in my lifetime, but Strecker was something else.

I asked Frank what he thought of him. Frank, who can smell a rat a mile away, thought Strecker made perfect sense. That confused me all the more.

I hated to admit it, but there was something about Strecker's unorthodox ideas that rang true. Even though there were plenty of missing details, I had a gut feeling he was onto something that merited investigation.

In a way I couldn't yet fully define, Strecker's beliefs prodded me to reexamine many questions that had bothered me since the beginning of the epidemic.

Where did the AIDS virus come from? Could it be man-made as Strecker suggested?

Why did it initially attack only gay men? Could they have been injected with the AIDS virus as Strecker proposed?

Why were central Africans and Haitians at "high-risk" for AIDS? Strecker also had the answer to that question.

Why did the scientific experts initially insist on calling AIDS a "gay" disease?

Why did they quickly separate AIDS from cancer?

Who were these AIDS experts? And how did they rapidly become experts of a disease most doctors knew little or nothing about?

Arriving home, I was exhausted. I tried to sleep, but my mind was still racing.

My anger deepened with every sleepless hour. I knew why. I hated thinking about Strecker's terrifying ideas which chilled my soul. The idea of a government plot to rid the nation of undesirables of one sort or another was mind-boggling!

I asked myself over and over again. Was the AIDS virus deliberately "introduced" into gay men in America?

Was there foul play in Africa? In Haiti?

Was my friend Gregg correct? Could the epidemic be a form of biological genocide?

Suppose Strecker was right, what was the evidence?

I remembered Strecker telling the group, "It's all in the scientific literature. You can find plenty of evidence for what I am saying in the medical libraries. All you have to do is take the time to look."

I had to know the truth. But where would I start?

Perhaps I could start with the first cases of AIDS that were discovered in gay men in Manhattan. I could reread the early AIDS literature. If there was foul play, surely there would be some clues.

There was no way medical science could perform a diabolic experiment of genocide, and get away with it. There was no way that could be.

I had to prove to myself that Strecker was wrong.

How could he know all this stuff that no one else knew anything about? I felt like a fool. My ego was shattered. I had prided myself in knowing things about AIDS that few others knew. And here was Strecker not knowing anything about cancer bacteria and trying to convince me the AIDS epidemic was biological warfare.

I had done a tremendous amount of scientific work. To my satisfaction, I had solved the mystery of AIDS when I discovered "cancer bacteria." And now Strecker was attempting to solve the mystery of AIDS in a wholly different way.

Suddenly I had become involved in the ultimate horror story of all time. If true, Strecker's story of a deliberate biological attack on humanity was the most frightening and diabolic deed ever perpetrated on this planet.

I had stepped into a web of scientific insanity, and I instinctively knew there was no way I could untangle myself from it.

I had to find the truth.

With that decision, my mind finally quieted. I fell into a deep sleep, too exhausted to dream, not knowing that the nightmare had begun.

References:

Wuerthele-Caspe Livingston V: *Cancer, A New Break-through,* Nash Publishing Corporation, Los Angeles, 1972.

Livingston-Wheeler V, Addeo EG: *The Conquest of Cancer,* Franklin Watts, New York, 1985.

CHAPTER THREE

The Cancer Virologists and Their Mission

The discovery of the AIDS virus enabled the cancer virologists to become the new shamans of medical science in America. As a result, national and local policies on AIDS testing, surveillance, research, treatment, and prevention are greatly influenced by the scientific opinions of these award-winning AIDS virologists.

Closely allied to these virologists are the high-ranking epidemiologists, who are primarily employed by the U.S. Public Health Service, or by the country's most prestigious medical institutions. Working hand-in-hand with this coterie are the most powerful pharmaceutical companies in the nation.

In short, this clique now runs the war on AIDS.

Within less than a decade, certain members of this clique have risen from scientific obscurity to the heights of scientific prominence. Their collective achievements could not have been accomplished were it not for the burgeoning of the AIDS epidemic.

The ill-fated and forgotten War on Cancer which began in the early 1970s has been quietly and unceremoniously transformed into the new War on AIDS. IRONICALLY, MANY OF THE SAME SCIENTISTS

WHO FAILED TO FIND THE CAUSE AND THE CURE FOR HUMAN CANCER HAVE NOW BECOME THE NEW LEADERS IN THE ASSAULT AGAINST THE AIDS VIRUS.

The so-called War on Cancer officially began with the signing of the National Cancer Act by President Richard Nixon, on December 23, 1971. Nixon, along with a host of politicians, was determined to launch an all-out, government-supported scientific attack on cancer, which would finally put a stop to this dread disease. Officials were hopeful that a cancer cure would be discovered in time for America's bicentennial birthday celebration in 1976.

The first appointed director of the newly-established National Cancer Program was Frank Rauscher, a young virologist who was greatly admired by Nixon. With Rauscher at the helm, it was easy for research cancer virologists and immunologists to be pushed to the forefront of the government's War on Cancer.

Back in the 1950s the cancer virologists first began to promote seriously their idea that cancer was caused by viruses. But by the 1970s, virologists had failed to prove their theory. The idea of a "cancer virus" was still ignored by most doctors who had been carefully taught in medical school that cancer was not a contagious or an infectious disease. Despite the virologists and their animal cancer experiments, physicians remained steadfast in their belief that no virus caused cancer.

During the 1950s and 60s, most doctors also believed that the immune system had nothing to do with the cause, treatment, or prevention of cancer. However, with increasing use of cancer chemotherapy during the 1960s, doctors began to develop a new respect for immunologists and their contention that the immune system was important in the body's defense against cancer.

By the end of the 1970s, against overwhelming odds, the cancer virologists had pushed themselves to the forefront of medical science with the financial support of powerful government institutions, and the political pull of people like Rauscher. THE CANCER VIROLO-GISTS WERE DETERMINED TO PROVE THAT VIRUSES WERE INVOLVED IN HUMAN CANCER.

Unlike bacteria (which are easily seen microscopically), viruses are too tiny to be seen in the common light-microscope. Viruses can be visualized by use of the electron microscope which magnifies objects 100,000 times or more, although it is often techically difficult to identify viruses in infected cells. The study of viruses is further complicated by the fact that viruses (unlike bacteria) grow only *inside* living cells.

It is also difficult to infect laboratory animals with certain viruses. Some inoculated viruses take a long time to produce disease effects in animals. In the past, animal inoculation experiments were often ruined because the animals frequently died of *other* causes before the virus experiment was over.

During the late 1950s, the ability to grow and study viruses was greatly stimulated by the new technique of laboratory tissue cell culture. Viruses could be seeded onto glass tubes containing sheets of live cells. For the first time, virologists could directly observe the effects of virus infection on living cells.

Amazingly, some new tissue culture "cell lines" proved

to be "immortal." If fed properly by lab technicians, the cells could continue to live and multiply indefinitely.

Tissue cell culture techniques brought revolutionary changes (as well as havoc) into the field of cancer-virus research, as chronicled in Michael Gold's *A Conspiracy of Cells*, (1986).

The history of human tissue cell culture began with Henrietta Lacks, a young black woman from Baltimore, who died from a highly malignant cervical cancer in 1951. Despite radiation and surgery, and the valiant attempt of the doctors to save her, Henrietta's cervical tumor spread rapidly throughout her body. Within eight months, she was dead.

But part of Henrietta's cancer remained alive. During her cancer surgery, some small pieces of the malignant tumor were donated to a laboratory which specialized in tissue cell culture. In those days, tissue culturing was a frustrating business. Most attempts to grow human cells outside the body failed. Rarely, a few cells would thrive for a while, and then die off.

For some unknown reason, Henrietta's cancer cells continued to grow vigorously. Her malignant cells eventually became the first successful human tissue culture "cell line" in medical history — the now famous "*HeLa*" cell line commemorating the legendary *HE*nrietta *LA*cks.

Henrietta's cancer cells were kept alive by feeding them a concoction that seemed more like a witches' brew than a laboratory recipe for cell culture. Nevertheless, the success of the recipe heralded a new age of modern virology.

According to Michael Gold, the laboratory concoction which fed Henrietta's cancer cells consisted of:

1. blood from human placentas (the placenta is the sac that nurtures the developing fetus. It also contains powerful hormones and a host of viruses and bacteria, as yet not fully investigated)
2. beef embryo extract (the ground-up remains of a three-week- old, unborn cattle embryo)
3. fresh chicken plasma obtained from the blood of a live chicken heart.

I wondered how many chicken, cattle, and human viruses were incorporated into Henrietta's immortal cancer cells by the chicken-beef-and human blood and tissue concoction that fed her cells. But none of this seemed to bother the virologists and the microbiologists. Undoubtedly, they have great faith that HeLa cells are free of all infectious agents.

All this aside, not only did Henrietta's cells thrive on this mixture but the live tissue culture proved so hardy that when it was passed around to laboratory investigators over the next few decades, the "immortal" HeLa cell line frequently contaminated other tissue culture cell lines used in cancer and cancer virus research.

In the late 1960s, when widespread HeLa cell contamination of cell lines was uncovered, scientists were shocked and embarrassed to learn that millions of dollars worth of published cancer research experiments were ruined. "Liver cells" and "monkey cells" that were used in cancer experiments turned out to be Henrietta's cervical cancer cells in disguise. Benign cells, which suddenly "spontaneously transformed" into malignant cells, were retrospectively found to be cell cultures which had been inadvertantly contaminated with HeLa.

In the late 1970s and 1980s, some published "discoveries" of "new" human cancer and AIDS-like viruses turned out to be "old" contaminant viruses in disguise.

As was the case with HeLa cell contamination, a conspiracy of silence surrounds the ever-present problem of virus contamination in cancer research. One notable example was the isolation of a "new" human retrovirus, "HL23," which was cultured from human leukemia cells. The "new" virus was later discovered to be not one, but two "old" contaminating monkey viruses.

Few people outside the field of virology know about these serious virus contamination problems. Could the AIDS epidemic have been started by a laboratory virus that inadvertantly "got out?" Could AIDS have been first "introduced" into American gays and black Africans through vaccine programs contaminated with AIDS-like monkey viruses? — and then "covered-up" by blaming the epidemic on African green monkeys?

With AIDS, the virologists had seemingly proved that human viruses caused cancer. But there were people, like Strecker and me, who had serious doubts. There was no question that viruses (and bacteria) could be isolated and grown from some cancer tumors, but were these cancer viruses the cause of cancer, or were they the effect? Did viruses really initiate cancer, or did the cancerous cell somehow attract and "pick-up" the viruses? It was the old "which came first story" — the chicken or the egg?

The problem with animal and human cancer viruses was that many of them were "exogenous" in nature. They were not viruses that animals and people normally carried in their bodies. They had to be "acquired." They did not exist in nature; they had to be created in virus laboratories. Strecker and I were amazed to read that some virologists freely admit that cancer viruses are basically laboratory artifacts.

In addition, it is very difficult to isolate cancer viruses from animals. A few cancer viruses can be grown, but only from certain cancer tumors that occur primarily in inbred and immunodeficient laboratory animals.

Some cancer-causing viruses are artificially produced. They often cause cancer and death when injected into animals, but that is still not proof that they cause cancer naturally.

Although all these experiments attempt to "prove" that viruses cause cancer in animals, it is obvious to critics that cancer is *never* produced that way in nature.

Putting aside HeLa cell contamination, as well as other major difficulties of cancer virus research, the biggest challenge the virologists faced in the early 1970s was to prove beyond doubt that viruses were the cause of *human* cancer. Unfortunately, despite years of research at the cost of millions of dollars, they still had not provided clear-cut evidence to prove the link between viruses and human cancer. And time was running out quickly.

The mounting frustration of the cancer virologists was apparent when they convened at a conference at Asilomar, near Pacific Grove, in Northern California in 1973. The conference, entitled "Biohazards in Biological Research," was sponsored by the world-renowned Cold Spring Harbor Laboratory, located at Cold Spring Harbor, New York.

Participating at the meeting were representatives from the most powerful government institutions, the top-ranking medical universities, and the most influential drug companies in the nation. The Asilomar conference was composed of the best and the brightest cancer virologists in America.

The biohazard problem in medical science was a serious subject. Many of the attending scientists were directors of the most sophisticated virus labs in America; laboratories that were designed for the study and manufacture of cancer viruses.

There were many dangers connected with these facilities. Not only were personnel heavily exposed to known viruses, but they were also exposed to newly-created and dangerous viruses that were synthesized in these virus laboratories.

The cancer reseachers coaxed all sorts of viruses into laboratory cell cultures. In addition, various viruses were injected or fed into animals for the sole purpose of producing cancer, immunodeficiency, opportunistic infections, and a host of other fatal diseases.

New diseases were produced in animals by viruses that were forced to "jump" from one species to another. Scientists put chicken viruses into lamb kidney cells. Baboon viruses were spliced into human cancer cells. Monkey viruses were grown in human blood cells. Ape leukemia viruses were inoculated into rat tissue cells. The combinations were endless.

But despite all this biogenetic cancer experimentation, there was still no solid proof that viruses caused cancer in human beings.

Robert Miller of the NCI emphasized this fact when

he addressed his colleagues: "Is cancer induced by viruses in man? Studies conducted to date have not implicated any virus. . . we simply do not have the epidemiologic methods to demonstrate that there is any cancer in man induced by a virus."

Others at the conference were more optimistic. Philip Cole, an epidemiologist at the Harvard School of Public Health, was convinced that careful scientific experiments combined with top-rate epidemiologic studies could prove a virus-cancer connection.

Cole envisioned two kinds of epidemiologic studies that could be done in tandem: a "retrospective" and a "prospective" cohort study. ("Cohort" is an epidemiologic term for a well-defined and carefully selected group of people who can be studied for statistical purposes).

A "retrospective" study could be made of a group of people *previously exposed* to a suspected cancer-causing virus. The "normal" and "expected" cancer disease rates for the cohort could be determined from statistics compiled by cancer tumor registries. If the "exposed" group developed a high rate of a certain kind of cancer, it would certainly suggest a cause-and-effect relationship between the virus and the cancer.

A "prospective" study could involve a cohort which *might be exposed* to a certain cancer virus *"in the future."* The group could be initially tested *before the exposure* and then "followed" into the future. At intervals, the cohort members would donate blood specimens for viral antibody study. These blood samples could be stored and tested from time to time. By testing the blood samples before-and-after the cancer virus exposure, the epidemiologists could determine when the infection occurred.

These necessary epidemiologic studies would also require a "surveillance system," as well as a central bureau which would be responsible for reporting the cancer incidence and the cancer deaths within the cohorts.

Cole stressed two points.

First, "the epidemiologic studies must not necessarily be limited to (virus) laboratory workers."

Cole's second point bears emphasis. "The epidemiologic studies which I have described could, especially if positive, have implications reaching far beyond our own health. Clearly, they would comprise ONE OF THE STRONGEST ARGUMENTS AVAILABLE THAT VIRUSES CAN CAUSE HUMAN CANCER (emphasis added). . . In any event, I can think of no more valuable epidemiologic studies which could be done now to evaluate the possible association between human cancer and horizontally transmitted oncogenic (cancer) viruses."

(Within less than a decade, Cole's vision became a reality when the hepatitis B gay cohorts were transformed into the epidemiologic model for AIDS in America. Cole's institution, the Harvard School of Public Health, would play a major role in the discovery of the AIDS virus, as well as in the discovery of "new" human and monkey AIDS retroviruses in Africa).

The Asilomar conference was geared to risky business. Michael Oxman of Harvard Medical School spoke on the potential biohazards of virus biological research. "Most of us will have to erect some barriers to protect ourselves, and others, from our experiments. . . and recognize the risks when such barriers are breached, either by infection *via unnatural routes, or as a consequence of physical or genetic alterations of the virus*. . . Personal ambition may convince an investigator to take certain risks."

Scientists like Francis Black of Yale University Medical School seemed willing to take risks. He declared, "If we do believe in our mission of trying to control cancer, it behooves us to accept some risk. Even if, as has been suggested, five or ten people might lose their lives, this might be a small price for the number of lives that would be saved."

At the conclusion of the meeting, the research scientists agreed to initiate "surveillance procedures" in case of a future "escape" of one of their deadly viruses into the environment. The establishment of a surveillance system and a central bureau would provide the vital epidemiologic data the virologists needed to fulfill their desperate mission to prove that viruses caused human cancer.

As I read the Proceedings of the Asilomar conference, I searched in vain for questions that were never raised by any of the brilliant scientists who collectively controlled the health of our nation.

It was apparent the experimental laboratories were not entirely safe. WHAT WOULD THE EXPERTS DO TO STOP A DEADLY VIRUS ONCE IT LEAKED OUT OF ONE OF THEIR HIGH-TECH LABORATORIES? WHAT WOULD THEY DO TO PROTECT THE PUBLIC FROM A NEW AND DEADLY DISEASE CAUSED BY A GENETICALLY ENGINEERED CANCER VIRUS THAT COULD SWIFTLY WIPE OUT LARGE NUMBERS OF PEOPLE?

Sadly, there were no answers to questions like these because no one raised them. The scientists only seemed interested in their "mission" to prove, once and for all, that their laboratory viruses could cause cancer in human beings.

By 1976, time was running out for the virologists and the War on Cancer. The politicians were not pleased with the virologists and their inability to come up with the promised cause or cure for cancer. Political pressure was put on Rauscher to step down, and he resigned in November 1976.

In 1977, Arthur Upton, an environmentalist, was appointed the new Director of the National Cancer Program. Under Upton's leadership, the new emphasis on cancer research would be the evaluation of environmental factors in cancer. From now on, the role of viruses in cancer would be downplayed.

By 1978, the cohorts of gay men had formed under the watchful eye of the government scientists. In November, the hepatitis B experimental vaccine trials began in Manhattan, New York City.

All the gay volunteers were young and healthy. They were perfect subjects for the experiment. They were specifically chosen because of their promiscuity and their lifestyle, and they were very cooperative. And they would be kept under strict "surveillance" by the government scientists and epidemiologists.

In 1979, physicians in Manhattan began to notice a new and deadly illness in young and previously healthy homosexual men. Many died pitifully of overwhelming infections. Peculiar, purple skin cancer blotches of Kaposi's sarcoma appeared on their faces and bodies.

This new kind of cancerous "scarlet letter" marked these men as perverts dying of an invariably fatal disease.

With the horrible deaths of thousands of gay men and other unfortunates, the scientists had the proof they so desperately required to fulfill their mission.

Quite accidentally, a strange new virus of unknown origin had been "introduced" into young gay men. Remarkably, the new virus could cause cancer — and immunodeficiency — and opportunistic infection — and death.

THE STRANGE VIRUS IN GAYS PERFORMED EXACTLY LIKE THE CANCER VIRUSES THAT WERE INJECTED INTO COUNTLESS NUMBERS OF FRIGHTENED AND SCREAMING ANIMALS CAGED IN CANCER LABORATORIES. It was quite a coincidence; a fortuitous and serendipitous happening. The "mission" of the virologists was accomplished. And they had done nothing to achieve it. The AIDS virus was an unfortunate accident of nature; a virus out of Africa that simply "jumped" species from green monkeys into man.

Quite by accident, the government epidemiologists had a perfect "model" in the cohorts of gay men that had formed at the request of the government for the hepatitis B experiment. The plan that had been hypothetically outlined years before at Asilomar had come to pass, mysteriously.

The young Manhattan gays were the perfect "retrospective" and the perfect "prospective" cohort needed to prove the "cancer-virus" connection. Since the mid-70s, thousands of other gay men had also been under "surveillance" in a number of large American cities. All these gays would serve well the experimental needs of the cancer virologists and the government epidemiologists.

The epidemiologists had the gay blood specimens neatly drawn. They had recorded the mens' names and addresses which would enable the epidemiologists to "follow" the men "into the future." And the gays were cooperating nicely by donating additional blood specimens every three to six months.

When the AIDS epidemic broke out in Manhattan, the hepatitis B gay cohort was quickly transformed into an AIDS cohort. This cohort, along with other government-established hepatitis B gay cohorts in San Francisco, Los Angeles, and other large American cities, proved to be the perfect epidemiological models to track the spread of the AIDS virus from gay men to the rest of the population.

With time, the hepatitis B cohorts would be transformed into cohorts of death.

THE RAPID DISCOVERY OF THE AIDS VIRUS WAS UNPRECEDENTED IN THE HISTORY OF MODERN MEDICAL SCIENCE. The new "gay plague" proved beyond doubt that viruses caused cancer and immunodepression.

In 1984, all this was a tremendous revelation to medical doctors, most of whom had erroneously believed that AIDS was caused by the cytomegalovirus (CMV). Their error was understandable. CMV was a sexually-transmitted virus found in body fluids. CMV infection was rampant in promiscuous gays, and was transmitted in semen.

At the beginning of the epidemic the doctors had been told by the expert virologists, immunologists and epidemiologists, that CMV was the most likely cause of AIDS. With the discovery of the AIDS virus, the previous statistics and epidemiologic evidence implicating cytomegalovirus as the cause of AIDS was suddenly out of fashion. From now on, the government scientists would carefully teach the physicians all they needed to know about the "new" virus and the "new" epidemic it was causing.

Strecker insisted the virologists and immunologists knew the real "origin" of the AIDS virus all along. It would be impossible for them not to know. The results of viral experiments published in the early 70s in their virology journals had proved that animal cancer viruses could cause cancer, immune depression, and opportunistic infection. To savvy retrovirologists, the brilliant "new" AIDS discoveries of the 80s were an obvious rehash of the decade-old science of animal cancer retrovirus experimentation.

For all their supposed brilliance, the best and the brightest scientists didn't have the foggiest idea how to stop the AIDS virus now that it was "introduced" into human beings. But none of this should have been surprising to those who were aware of the nature of the animal cancer experiments that epitomized the War on Cancer.

After all, the primary purpose of these animal and cell experiments was to create cancer with tiny genetic packages of death. Nobody was demanding that these same scientists learn to heal cancer. That was not their task.

Strecker insisted I learn more about the cancer experts. It seemed a good idea. Although many of the AIDS experts rarely held the hand of a dying AIDS patient, they seemed to know a lot about AIDS that I didn't.

I wondered how they got so damn smart so quickly.

References:

Karpas A, Maayan S, Raz R: Lack of antibodies to adult T-cell leukemia virus and to AIDS virus in Israeli Falashas. Nature 319: 794, 1986.

Gold M: *A Conspiracy of Cells*, State University of New York Press, Albany, 1986.

Biohazards in Biological Research, Cold Spring Harbor Laboratory, Cold Spring Harbor, New York, 1973.

Moss RW: *The Cancer Syndrome*, Grove Press Inc, New York, 1980.

CHAPTER FOUR

The Animal Experimenters and AIDS

The Albert Lasker Medical Research Award is the most prestigious scientific award offered in America. But it is much more than that. Winning a Lasker Award is often a prelude to receiving the world's most coveted honor: the Nobel prize. Sooner or later, over 65% of Lasker winners get a Nobel Prize for their scientific achievements.

In 1986 the Lasker award was presented to three distinguished scientists: Myron (Max) Essex, Robert Gallo, and Luc Montagnier. All three men were instrumental in discovering the cause of AIDS — the so-called AIDS virus.

Essex and Gallo's award-winning achievements were a perfect example of how the experimental production of cancer and immunodepression in animals could provide the key to understanding a new and still-mysterious epidemic disease of cancer and immunodepression.

A careful perusal of their scientific research during the 1970s, explains how the experimental inoculation of laboratory animals with cancer viruses eventually led to the discovery of the AIDS virus in gay men.

Max Essex is a veterinarian; a doctor trained in the study and treatment of animal diseases. He is professor of virology, and chairman of the Department of Cancer Biology at the Harvard School of Public Health.

In a series of cat experiments performed during the 1970s, Essex attempted to prove that feline (cat) leukemia was caused by a cancer-inducing virus. By the end of the decade, his research indicated that cat leukemia was caused by a specific RNA retrovirus. This cancer-causing, AIDS-like virus was named feline leukemia virus (FeLV).

Essex's cat experiments provided the first scientific evidence that A CANCER-CAUSING VIRUS COULD BE CONTAGIOUS, AND COULD CAUSE SUPPRESSION OF THE IMMUNE SYSTEM!

Details of these experiments are worth reviewing because they help to explain how a veterinarian could garner world-renowned honors for solving the AIDS puzzle, along with Gallo and Montagnier.

One experiment involved ten 4 month-old kittens who had never been exposed to feline leukemia virus (FeLV). The kittens (called "tracers" in the experiment) were placed in a house with other cats who had already been infected with the virus.

The blood of the young "tracer" cats was tested frequently during the experiment to determine if they had been infected with FeLV. Within 18 months, seven of the ten tracer cats died (3 developed aplastic anemia, 3 infectious peritonitis, and 1 lymphoma). The FeLV could be isolated from the blood of all seven. The remaining three cats stayed healthy, but their blood developed high-titer antibodies to FeLV.

Essex's experiment, reported in 1977, "clearly indicated that unprotected post-weanling cats brought into a leukemia exposure household environment have a high risk of becoming infected with FeLV."

Another report, published in 1979, involved the study of 184 cats with leukemia and lymphoma. (Clinically, these two types of cat cancer are indistinguishable from one another). Two-thirds of the cancerous cats were virus-positive for FeLV; one-third were virus-negative. The actual cause of the tumors in the virus-negative cats was not clear, but the researchers were convinced that these cancers were caused by FeLV.

The results of another important "Cat house" experiment were published in 1980. During the years 1972-1977, scientists studied a group of 134 cats living in a 10-room house in Connecticut. All the cats eventually became infected with FeLV virus and carried antibodies to the virus in their blood. However, only 54% of the cats carried "live" FeLV in their blood. These "viremic" cats had a much higher mortality rate (a factor of 34.6 versus 8.9) than the non-viremic cats who did not carry the live virus. Most cats died from kidney disease (glomerulonephritis) and lymphoma cancer.

After a decade of feline cancer research, Essex and his colleagues concluded that feline leukemia/lymphoma was caused by FeLV. Cat leukemia was the most thoroughly investigated example of a naturally occurring *"community acquired"* infection due to a cancer-causing virus. It was predicted that similar cancer viruses might be the cause of some human cancers, especially the leukemia/lymphoma type of cancer.

Within two years of this 1980 report, epidemiologists would be declaring that AIDS was THE FIRST (HOMOSEXUAL) "COMMUNITY ACQUIRED" EPIDEMIC OF IMMUNODEPRESSION AND CANCER THAT HAD EVER BEEN RECORDED IN MEDICAL HISTORY.

In the early days of the epidemic, some virologists believed there was a similarity in the way feline leukemia, hepatitis B, and AIDS were all transmitted. A 1981 report by Max Essex, Donald Francis (who had worked in Essex's lab), and James Maynard compared the cat leukemia/lymphoma viruses with hepatitis B virus in terms of their ability to cause cancer. For example, they stressed that FeLV could lead to leukemia and lymphoma cancer in cats, while hepatitis B virus could lead to liver cancer in human beings.

But despite all the cat cancer studies, the general scientific community was still skeptical about the role of any virus in human cancer.

The cancer virologists and the animal experimenters were frustrated. They were absolutely convinced that retroviruses could cause human cancer.

Francis, Essex, and Maynard wrote: "There are many similarities between infections caused by FeLV in cats and hepatitis B virus in humans. . . The uniqueness of such virus-induced human cancer should not mean that the scientific community should be dismayed by and reluctant to believe the association. . . On the contrary, it fits the patterns that might be expected for a naturally-occurring oncogenic virus and should serve to. . . stimulate the search for other similar agents in humans."

In early 1983, (more than a year before the official "discovery" of the AIDS virus), the Editors of the *Journal of the National Cancer Institute* solicited a "guest editorial" on AIDS from Essex, Francis, and James Curran (from the CDC in Atlanta). Officials at the National Cancer Institute were convinced that AIDS would increase their understanding of cancer.

As proof of this, The Editor of the *Journal* noted: "Periodically, the *Journal* publishes solicited guest editorials as a means of transmitting to investigators in cancer research the essence of current work in a special field of study. The Board of Editors welcomes suggestions for future editorials that succinctly summarize current work toward *a clearly defined hypothesis regarding the causes and cure of cancer.*"

The July 1983 Editorial was entitled "Epidemic AIDS: Epidemiologic evidence for a transmissible Agent." Francis, Essex, and Curran wrote with confidence about their understanding of AIDS: "An infectious agent, presumably a virus, is the most likely etiologic candidate. . . Some animal viruses share epidemiologic and clinical characteristics with this presumed agent. A review of these two viruses, Hepatitis B virus and FeLV of cats might help elucidate the etiology of this disease and help direct research."

They continued with their intimate knowledge of feline leukemia/lymphoma, the profound implications of which were known to very few medical doctors at the time. (In 1983, as noted earlier, most physicians erroneously believed that the cytomegalovirus was the most likely cause of AIDS). "FeLV, an RNA virus of the retrovirus genus, replicates in multiple tissues and produces persistent viremia; IT CAUSES CANCER AND IMMUNOSUPPRESION in cats through its effects on lymphocytes. . . Three major categories of disease are associated with chronic FeLV—OPPORTU-NISTIC INFECTIONS, IMMUNE COMPLEX DIS-EASE, AND CANCER. . . The cancers caused by this virus are most commonly leukemias and lymphomas."

Donald Francis, (who had supervised the hepatitis B vaccine experimental trials in gay men in five American cities), emphasized that "the epidemiologic similarities between hepatitis B virus and the putative AIDS agent are striking. . . and (hepatitis B virus) shares many similarities with RNA tumor viruses such as FeLV."

Eight months *before* this July 1983 Editorial, Robert Gallo, a cancer retrovirologist, observed the AIDS virus in white blood cell lymphocytes at the National Cancer Institute. This may explain why the three scientists wrote so confidently about the "hypothetical AIDS virus."

In April 1984, Gallo solved the AIDS mystery. His quick discovery of the AIDS virus would not have been possible without the help of his friend and collaborator, Max Essex, who supplied Gallo with some badly-needed technological supplies and know-how.

As Essex and his cat experiments with the feline leukemia/lymphoma virus faded into the background, Gallo came to the fore with his new AIDS "leuke-mia/lymphoma" virus. Immediately, Gallo began to weave complex and elaborate theories to explain the African origin of the AIDS virus.

Who was Robert Gallo, and how was he able to solve

the mystery of AIDS so quickly?

As a young boy of 13, Gallo painfully watched his younger sister die from leukemia. This experience must have influenced him to become a physician, and to devote his life to cancer research. In 1965, he joined the staff of the National Cancer Institute, and began his landmark studies in leukemia research in 1970.

Gallo was the first to discover an enzyme called reverse transcriptase in cancerous leukemia cells. This enzyme was produced by retroviruses, and Gallo had a strong hunch retroviruses might be the cause of leukemia.

In 1978, he became the first scientist to discover and isolate a human retrovirus from malignant T-cells in the blood of a cancer patient.

This spectacular achievement was made possible by new advances in virology and immunology, such as better purification of viral proteins, newer nucleic acid probes, and the development of monoclonal and hyperimmune antibodies.

Gallo named his cancer retrovirus HUMAN T-CELL *LEUKEMIA/LYMPHOMA* VIRUS, or "HTLV-1" for short.

HTLV-1 is the prototype of a "family" of human retroviruses. Later, when other similar-appearing viruses were discovered, Gallo included them in his HTLV "family" of viruses.

Beginning in 1977, reports out of Japan indicated that a new illness resembling leukemia and lymphoma was being recognized in southwestern Japan, especially on the island of Kyushu. The illness was called "adult T-cell leukemia" (ATL). The leukemia cases occurred in clusters; and the Japanese strongly suspected a "new" virus was causing the disease.

Based on his prior investigations of leukemia, Gallo believed the new disease might also be caused by one of his HTLV-type cancer viruses, and he set out to prove it. It was a perfect opportunity.

By this time (1981), Gallo's lab had perfected a technique to keep T-cells alive by adding a protein hormone called TCGF (T-cell growth factor) to the cell culture. Before TCGF, it was exceedingly difficult, if not impossible, to keep T-cells alive long enough to culture the infecting viruses growing within them. With TCGF the cells grew vigorously, enabling Gallo to capture and culture the infecting virus.

The new and exciting leukemia/lymphoma reports from Japan were the impetus that sparked an international conference in Kyoto in March 1981. The meeting was attended by top virologists and cell biologists from Japan, China, Korea, the United States and France.

Prior to the meeting, the Japanese sent Gallo blood samples from their leukemia/lymphoma patients. He shone at the Kyoto meeting by reporting the successful growth of a new virus (with the help of TCGF) from the leukemic blood cells. The virus was identical to Gallo's HTLV-1 virus that he had first discovered in an American patient with leukemia in 1978. Gallo detected his virus in almost 100% of the Japanese blood samples.

Where did the "new" Japanese-type HTLV virus come from? The virologists had no idea.

Three months after the Kyoto meeting, the American public first learned of a "new" epidemic disease that had started in homosexuals in New York City. A year later, "AIDS" became a household word.

The experts studying the new epidemic wondered where the mysterious immunosuppressive agent of AIDS could have come from. No one knew for sure.

In the early 1980s, another cluster of leukemia/ lymphoma cases was discovered in Caribbean blacks. The cases were similar to those found in southern Japan, on the island of Kyushu. In Gallo's lab, an HTLV virus was grown from the T-cells of the Caribbean blacks. It looked and acted just like the Japanese virus.

Could these new HTLV viruses be related to known animal viruses and retroviruses? A 1982 report on the Caribbean cases written by Gallo, Blattner, *et al* emphasized that the new HTLV virus in blacks was NOT closely related to any known animal retrovirus. However, another 1982 paper on HTLV co-authored by Oroszlan, Gallo, *et al* suggested that "HTLV MAY BE CLOSER TO BOVINE (CATTLE) LEUKEMIA THAN ANY OTHER KNOWN RETROVIRUS." (This seemed to confirm Strecker's concept of the similarity of the AIDS virus to the bovine leukemia virus).

In another 1982 paper, Gallo (in collaboration with another scientist from UCLA) reported the discovery of a "second" HTLV virus in the T-cells of a patient with a rare form of leukemia, known as "hairy cell leukemia." The new virus was closely related to HTLV-1, but not identical. Gallo named the virus HTLV-2.

In August 1982, Gallo was appointed Director of AIDS research at NCI. And he was again determined to prove that AIDS was caused by one of his HTLV viruses.

With the help of Max Essex from Harvard, he began to test the blood of 75 AIDS patients for HTLV antibodies. Surprisingly, HTLV-1 antibodies were found in 25% of the blood samples.

By 1983, Gallo's AIDS research seemed the most promising of all, and the media and the medical reporters kept close tabs on his views. In a 1983 *JAMA* interview, a reporter asked Gallo why he was looking for HTLV in AIDS.

He answered, "First, it's intriguing that the family we call HTLV is quite new in certain populations. HTLV was really discovered only five years ago; AIDS is also a new disease. Second, some retroviruses are known in animals to be capable of causing not only leukemias or lymphoma but also severe immunosuppression. FELINE LEUKEMIA VIRUS, A RETROVIRUS QUITE SIMILAR TO HTLV, IS AN EXAMPLE. Generally speaking, immune suppression is a hallmark of AIDS." Gallo reminded the reporter that his "laboratory was particularly well equipped methodologically to detect this kind of virus."

During the 20 months that Gallo informally collaborated with Essex, the development of a sensitive immunologic test to detect low-levels of HTLV virus was perfected. The preliminary results suggested that another kind of HTLV virus was involved in AIDS. This strange virus shared some similar properties with HTLV-1 and HTLV-2, but there were DISTINCT GENETIC STRUCTURAL DIFFERENCES OF THE AIDS VIRUS WHICH DISTINGUISHED IT FROM HTLV-1 AND HTLV-2.

At a press conference held on April 23, 1984, Gallo

declared to the scientific world that he and his co-workers at NCI had discovered the virus that caused AIDS.

Where did the new virus come from? This time there would be an answer. The media and the science writers listened attentively and reported every word Gallo spoke.

According to *TIME* magazine (April 30, 1984), Gallo claimed the new HTLV-3 strain of the AIDS virus evolved in Africa. "The virus may have been around in the bush for some time, but with mass migration into cities, crowding and prostitution, what was contained at a low level became a problem."

NEWSWEEK (May 7, 1984) pictured a world map showing arrows pointing to probable routes of the AIDS virus "on the move" out of central Africa. The accompanying description read:

1. "AIDS probably appeared first in Africa, as the result of a minor genetic change in a less lethal virus, or when rural people who harbored the virus moved to urban areas.
2. French and Belgians who lived in central Africa presumably carried the disease back to Western Europe. AIDS also traveled to the Caribbean, possibly brought there by Haitians.
3. From Haiti, vacationing homosexuals from the United States may have brought AIDS home."

Gallo had fulfilled his goal. But there was one big problem. The French scientists were declaring that *they* had discovered the cause of AIDS one year before Gallo. They claimed they deserved the recognition, not he. The French contingent was headed by Luc Montagnier, and he was determined the French should get the scientific recognition and the rewards they so rightfully deserved — and, if necessary, they would go to court to get it.

Scientists rarely work alone. To be accepted, their work must be reported in peer-reviewed scientific journals where it can be carefully scrutinized by other investigators. There is also big money to be made from the new epidemic, especially for researchers and for drug companies who know how to get the most profit out of scientific discoveries as earth-shattering as the AIDS virus. The patent on the AIDS blood testing kits which will be used by countless numbers of people throughout the world is worth millions of dollars.

Pharmaceutical companies that come up with a vaccine or a drug to fight AIDS will amass a fortune. In short, AIDS is big business for the medical and drug industry.

Early in the epidemic in 1982, French scientists had a problem that forced them into AIDS research and into the AIDS economy. A French company wanted to release the new commercial hepatitis B preventive vaccine, but there was fear the vaccine might have some connection with AIDS (or SIDA, as it is called in France). Luc Montagnier was called upon to try to determine whether a virus was involved in this new mystery disease.

Montagnier was head of cancer virology at the Pasteur Institute in Paris, the most famous medical research establishment in the world. Along with other

Pasteur scientists, Montagnier was familiar with the latest American advances in cancer virology; and discoveries and information were freely shared between American and French scientists.

In January 1983, Montagnier and his colleagues isolated a retrovirus from an enlarged lymph node of a young gay Frenchman with "early" symptoms of AIDS. Not surprisingly, the man had visited New York City in 1979. (In 1987, the man was still alive and healthy). The Pasteur Institute researchers knew their strange retrovirus had some similarity to HTLV. They called upon Gallo to help them identify their virus, and Gallo agreed.

According to Marlene Cimons (*Los Angeles Times Magazine*, May 25, 1986), the French virus wouldn't grow in Gallo's lab, and it was pigeon-holed. Nevertheless, the French kept working on identifying their virus, convinced that it had something to do with AIDS. They named the virus "lymphadenopathy virus" (LAV), and they wrote a scientific report on their laboratory findings.

Prior to the publication of this research in *Science* magazine, the scientific paper was sent to Gallo for revisions and comments. Gallo suggested the French virus appeared to be a member of his HTLV "family" of viruses.

Montagnier's French report, complete with pictures of the French "lymphadenopathy virus" (LAV), was published in the May 1983 issue of *Science*. (*LAV eventually was proven to be "the" AIDS virus*). The same issue of *Science* also contained two papers by Gallo, and another by Essex. The independent studies of all three researchers pointed to a new virus as the probable cause of AIDS.

Montagnier's paper was largely ignored by the scientists, who preferred to believe that Gallo and Essex's work was closer to the truth. They were undoubtedly influenced by Gallo who was not exactly sure Montagnier's group had found the "true" virus of AIDS.

The CDC was even more unkind in their appraisal of LAV. In the CDC *Morbidity and Mortality Weekly Report* (May 13, 1983), the French virus was declared "clearly distinct" from HTLV. (Two years later, LAV and HTLV-3 were found to be "almost identical").

In April 1984, Gallo officially announced his new virus was the cause of AIDS. The discovery was heralded by the top scientists in government. Overnight, the physicians became believers in the new AIDS virus.

The following year, the private bickering between the French and the American AIDS scientists became front-page news. The Pasteur Institute filed suit against the U.S. Federal Government. The lawsuit was not surprising. The royalties to the new HTLV-3 antibody test were worth millions, and the French wanted their share.

Gallo finally admitted the French had published the first paper on the AIDS virus, complete with pictures. With time, most scientists accepted the fact that LAV and HTLV-3 were as identical as any two AIDS viruses could be. It was also evident to me that *"clearly distinct"* viruses could turn out to be *"almost identical"* viruses. It all depended on the expert who was making the claim.

I was beginning to understand why I had such a hard time trying to understand virology and virologists. There was a lot of double talk going on, cleverly guised in scientific language that nobody but virologists could understand.

Gallo's anger with Montagnier was hardly a private matter. The *Los Angeles Times* (Dec 14, 1985) quoted him as saying: "They got the idea from us. . . I was the first to suggest it was a retrovirus. We had this virus in 1982. We didn't publish on purpose because we didn't understand it well enough to stick our necks out. To me *discovery* is a complicated word. Who first reported discovery of a virus? They did. But if the idea comes first — that was us."

Despite the animosity, the French and American scientists were rejoined in medical history when they each received their Lasker Awards for their contributions to the War against AIDS. Medical reporters noted their public bickering would not bode well with the Nobel Prize Committee. The Committee had a reputation of shunning scientists whose work provoked bad publicity, legal disputes, and malice. After all, the Nobel Prize was associated with purity in science, and the washing of dirty linen on the front pages of the leading world newspapers was very tacky.

With the discovery of the AIDS virus, the animal cancer-virus experiments of the 70s were quickly forgotten, along with the connection between hepatitis B and AIDS.

The short history of AIDS was filled with coincidences that were unprecedented in medical science. Instead of the clinical physicians, the veterinarians in animal cancer research and the cancer virologists were walking off with the AIDS research awards. The veterinarians and the cancer virologists were quickly transformed into the new AIDS experts.

The physician-epidemiologists, who had supervised the experimental hepatitis B vaccine trials in gay men in large American cities, were also catapulted to high positions in AIDS research.

Within a few short years the virologists had regained the glory that they had almost lost when they couldn't prove that human cancer was caused by a virus.

AIDS made the cancer retrovirologists the new shamans of medicine. They taught the doctors to believe that cancer could be caused by retroviruses. And the doctors believed without question. After all, the "official" word had come down from the establishment.

The deaths of thousands of gay men with AIDS had humbled the egos of medical doctors who were powerless to stop the deaths. The only hope for a future treatment and a cure for AIDS would have to come from these new shamans, all with their high-powered, official government connections.

And what about gay men? Why had they been marked for the first mass deaths from AIDS? Why had they so rapidly become the new human "experimental animals" for medical research?

How did the gays get drawn into the web of AIDS? Was it just a coincidence — a quirk of fate? Or was it deliberately planned?

References:

Essex M, Cotter SM, Sliski AH, et al: Horizontal transmission of feline leukemia virus under natural conditions in a feline leukemia cluster household. Int J Cancer 19:90-96, 1977.

Francis DP, Cotter SM, Hardy WD Jr, Essex M: Comparison of virus-positive and virus-negative cases of feline leukemia and lymphoma. Cancer Research 39:3899-3870, 1979.

Francis DP, Essex M, Jakowski RM, et al: Increased risk for lymphoma and glomerulonephritis in a closed population of cats exposed to feline leukemia virus. Amer J Epidemiology 111:377-346, 1980.

Francis DP, Essex M: Leukemia and lymphoma: Infrequent manifestations of common viral infections? A Review. J Infect Dis 138:916-923, 1978.

Francis DP, Essex M, Maynard JE: Feline leukemia virus and hepatitis B virus: A comparison of late manifestations. Prog Med Virol 27:127-132, 1981.

Francis DP, Curran JW, Essex M: Epidemic acquired immune deficiency syndrome: Epidemiological evidence for a transmissible agent. JNCI 71:1-4, 1983.

Gallo RC, de The GB, Ito Y: Kyoto workshop on some specific recent advances in human tumor virology. Cancer Research 41:4738-4739, 1981.

Blattner WA, Kalyanaraman VS, Robert-Guroff M,

Gallo RC, et al: The human type-C T-cell retrovirus, HTLV, in blacks from the Caribbean region, and relationship to adult T-cell leukemia. Int J Cancer 30:257-264, 1982.

Oroszlan S, Sarngadharan MG, Copeland TD, Gallo RC, et al: Primary structure analysis of the major internal protein p24 of human type-C T-cell leukemia virus. Proc Nat Acad Sci 79:1291-1294, 1982.

Maurice J: Human "T" Leukemia virus still suspected in AIDS. JAMA 250:1015,1021,1983.

CHAPTER FIVE

The Hepatitis B Vaccine Trials (1978-1981)

For most of this century, doctors have "classified" homosexuals as mentally ill people. Undoubtedly, this medical judgment against gay people was largely based on Judeo-Christian strictures against homosexuality that persist to this day. However, the facts of the matter clearly indicate that there was never any sound scientific evidence to show that homosexuality was a disease or a mental disorder.

The medical profession's erroneous classification of homosexuality as a mental illness is a striking example of how "scientific" people can damage and destroy lives through ignorance, hate, and religious intolerance. Sadly, this condemnation against gays still pervades society. As a result, many physicians, as well as the general public, continue to regard homosexuals as "sick" people.

Because of the religious, scientific, and legal condemnation of homosexuality, most gay men and women in America remained firmly closeted until recent years. It was only with the sweeping social changes of the 1960s that the gay community began to organize against this harsh judgment of society. In a decade of mass public protests characterized by the Black Civil Rights Movement, the Women's Liberation Movement, and the Anti-Vietnam War Movement, the spark of revolution also ignited the gay community against the oppression of "straight" society.

On the evening of June 28, 1969, the Gay Liberation Movement erupted violently during a police raid on a gay bar called "The Stonewall" in New York City. The bar, located on Christopher Street in the Greenwich Village section of Manhattan, was one of the most popular night spots for homosexual men.

In those days, senseless and unprovoked police raids on gay bars were commonplace. Frightened customers were rounded up at random, and hauled-off to police stations for booking. The names and addresses of the arrested homosexuals often appeared in the newspapers which also listed the charges of lewd conduct and other sexual offenses. In the process of this public exposure and humiliation (and the implication of mental illness), many careers and lives were irrevocably damaged.

For some unknown reason this particular raid on Stonewall turned into a brawl when police attempted to arrest groups of homosexual men. A mob scene developed when scores of angry men began to fight the police.

Word of the riot quickly spread throughout the Village. The following night over two-thousand well-organized and feisty gay men and women congregated on Christopher Street to protest police harassment. Defiant crowds of homosexuals lingered on the streets of the Village for several days, and authorities were fearful that more bloody riots would erupt. Finally, under the threat of more gay demonstrations and planned acts of civil disobedience, the New York City police department backed down.

For the first time in history, the success of Stonewall ignited a spirit among gay people, and the Gay Pride Movement was born. A decade later, the "gay plague" descended on Manhattan.

Under political pressure from gay activists in the early 1970s, the American Psychiatric Association finally removed the stigma of mental illness from gay people. Although gays are no longer "classified" as having a mental illness, the World Health Organization (WHO) continues to classify homosexuality as a psychiatric disorder.

(In 1987, the WHO was publicly accused of unleashing the AIDS epidemic in central Africa, as a result of its smallpox vaccine programs. However, there were no allegations that the WHO had any involvement in the AIDS outbreak in American gays.)

In the decade after Stonewall, the movement soared to unbelievable heights of gay political power and clout. By the late 1970s, gay liberation had brought tens of thousands of homosexual men and women out of the closet, and openly gay communities were flourishing in Greenwich Village, San Francisco, and West Hollywood.

Gay Pride parades in San Francisco, Los Angeles, and New York, were shown on TV screens throughout America. For the first time, "straight" Americans were forced to face the fact that most gay people appeared perfectly "normal" and happy. Gays were "out" and they weren't ever going back into the closet.

Millions of Americans did not welcome the forced entry of "queers," "faggots" and "dykes" into their living rooms and bedrooms. Some complained the country was rapidly turning into a modern-day Sodom and Gomorrah; and many parents feared for their children's safety against this new breed of pushy perverts.

The struggle for Gay Rights in the late 1970s brought about the inevitable anti-gay backlash symbolized by political groups such as the Moral Majority. To this day, the backlash persists in the form of the anti-gay Right Wing Movement, and in the deadly sport of "gay bashing" and "gay murder."

The Gay Civil Rights Movement reached its apogee in November 1978. It was a tumultuous month which began with the defeat of "Proposition 6" by California voters. The Proposition, if passed, would have barred gays from teaching in that state. But November ended in disaster with the assasination of Harvey Milk at City Hall in San Francisco.

A year earlier, in 1977, Harvey Milk had become the first openly-gay candidate to win election to the San Francisco Board of Supervisors. For gay people, Milk became the ultimate political symbol attesting to all that was admirable and achievable in the Gay Pride movement.

Also elected to the Board was Dan White, a former paratrooper and ex-policeman, an Irish Catholic, and a notorious homophobe. Harvey Milk and Dan White represented the two faces of San Francisco politics and lifestyles. Milk represented the aging Hippie and the gay Jewish liberal; White symbolized the macho, All-American, anti-gay conservative.

During the ensuing year the enmity and political

intrigues between the two supervisors culminated in White's cold-blooded murder of Harvey Milk and George Moscone, the straight mayor of San Francisco, at City Hall on the morning of November 27, 1978. The anti-gay sentiments whipped up for the November congressional elections undoubtedly contributed to Dan White's homophobic madness and murderous deeds.

At the beginning of November, the gays were at the height of their political power, but the murder of Milk was a bad omen.

In November 1978, the experimental hepatitis B vaccine trials began in Manhattan. And it was the beginning of the end for American gays.

Strecker's theory that the AIDS virus was introduced into gays via the hepatitis B vaccine trials sent shock waves of disbelief through me that could only be quelled by a serious inquiry into his accusation.

But there was an inner feeling or vague intuition that he was correct. On the other hand, I'm sure I would never have taken him seriously had I not studied AIDS carefully in my own research. I knew from personal experience that AIDS researchers were ignoring extremely important observations that were crucial to a deeper and more complete understanding of the epidemic.

There was a common bond between Strecker and me, in that we shared a mutual distrust of what passed for AIDS "science." The AIDS epidemic reeked of medical and scientific politics. For the first time in my life, I was ashamed of the scientific arrogance that pervaded the medical profession. I sensed the medical science of AIDS was turning into something akin to Nazi science. Of course, I couldn't prove it. It was only a gut feeling, and it was deeply disturbing.

In a passion that bordered on frenzy, I struggled through paper after paper, trying to learn as much as I could about cancer virology, animal cancer-virus experimentation, and the politics of the cancer establishment. Without that background knowledge, it was impossible to understand the profound significance of the hepatitis vaccine trials in gay people.

Strecker's concept that biological warfare was at the root of AIDS was terrifying, and what I read in Robert Harris and Jeremy Paxman's secret story of chemical and biological warfare, *A Higher Form of Killing* (1982), added immeasurably to the horror. This definitive book on biowarfare stands as a testimony of man's inhumanity to man, and should be required reading for all people interested in protecting the planet from this "higher form of killing."

There are few Americans who are even vaguely aware that the U.S. Army has a Biological and Chemical Warfare Department, located at Fort Detrick in Frederick, Maryland. Its detailed functions are largely unknown, but the little I did learn sent chills down my spine.

During the 1960s, the Army's biological warfare program was largely geared to DNA and "gene splicing" research. In the late 1960s, President Nixon renounced germ warfare, except for "medical defensive research." This "defensive" research continues to the present time, and primarily centers around vaccine development and the genetic enginering of infectious agents capable of infecting large masses of people.

UNDER ORDERS FROM PRESIDENT NIXON IN 1971, A LARGE PART OF THE ARMY'S BIOLOGICAL WARFARE UNIT WAS TRANSFERRED TO THE NATIONAL CANCER INSTITUTE (NCI).

With the transfer of the unit to NCI, the army's DNA and genetic engineering programs were coordinated into anti-cancer research and molecular biology programs. Litton Bionetics, a division of Litton industries, was privately contracted to run the operation.

THE ARMY'S DEPARTMENT OF BIOLOGICAL WARFARE ALREADY HAD A WELL-DOCUMENTED TRADITION OF EXPERIMENTATION ON HUMAN BEINGS. To think otherwise would be naive. In time of war, the function and purpose of the Department are to zero in on particular populations and to destroy them. Certain biowarfare weapons have been uniquely designed for the targeting and killing of specific ethnic ("ethno-specific") and racial groups.

There are close economic and political ties between the Army Department of Biological Warfare, the CIA, the CDC, the NCI, the NIH, the World Health Organization, and private industry groups such as Litton Industries. A carefully orchestrated and clandestine human biological warfare experiment sanctioned by one or more of these governmental agencies could easily escape the attention of an unsuspecting scientific community and the public-at-large. The combined military and political power of all these federal and private agencies staggers the imagination.

Secret human experiments conducted by the Army and the CIA during the 1950s have only recently come to light. For example, "in August 1977 the CIA admitted that there had been no less that 149 subprojects, including experiments to determine the effects of different drugs on human behavior, work on lie-detectors, hypnosis and electric shock, and the surreptitious delivery of drug-related materials. Forty-four colleges and universities had been involved, fifteen research foundations, twelve hospitals or clinics and three penal institutions" (*A Higher Form of Killing*, page 210).

There are undoubtedly hundreds of horror stories of U.S. military personnel and civilians who have been damaged or even killed by such experiments. In 1958, James B. Stanley, an Army sargeant, volunteered to test gas masks and protective clothing as part of a chemical warfare experiment. But the experiment was a decoy to hide the real (and secret) experiment in which Stanley was repeatedly given LSD, as well as injections, to test the drug's effects. He suffered severe mental effects which eventually destroyed his Army career and his marriage.

Incredibly he learned about the secret experiment almost twenty years later when the Army contacted him for "follow-up." Culminating a series of legal battles, the U.S. Supreme Court ruled in June, 1987, that Stanley (now aged 53) could not sue the military because it would "disrupt the military regime."

According to *American Medical News* (July 17, 1987), Justice William Brennan, one of the dissenting judges, wrote: "Serious violations of the constitutional rights of soldiers must be exposed and punished. Soldiers ought not to be asked to defend a Constitution indifferent to their essential human dignity." The ruling allows government officials to "violate the constitutional right of soldiers without fear of money damages." Brennan likened Stanley's case to the Nazi atrocities in World War II concentration camps.

When I compared Strecker's biowarfare theory of a "man-made AIDS virus" with the so-called "green monkey theory" that the AIDS experts were expounding, I had to admit it didn't seem any less plausable. And unlike the theories of the other scientists, Strecker insisted his theory could be proven by reading the scientific literature. I requested every scientific paper which related to the experimental hepatitis B vaccine trials in gays, and I began to study them carefully.

TO MY SURPRISE, I QUICKLY DISCOVERED THAT MUCH OF THE SCIENTIFIC KNOWLEDGE THAT HAS ACCUMULATED ON THE "SPREAD" OF AIDS IN AMERICA HAS COME FROM THE SURVEILLANCE AND BLOOD TESTING OF LARGE GROUPS OF GAY AND BISEXUAL MEN WHO VOLUNTEERED AS HUMAN TEST SUB- JECTS IN THE ORIGINAL HEPATITIS B VACCINE TRIALS WHICH TOOK PLACE IN SIX AMERICAN CITIES DURING THE YEARS 1978-1981.

Was it coincidental that those were the beginning years of the new mystery disease in gays, and the years just before AIDS became "official?"

The intense interest of the government scientists in the control and eradication of "gay" sexually-transmitted diseases led to the creation of a surveillance system for large numbers of gay people during the mid-1970s. This surveillance continues up to the present time in the form of cohorts of gay men who provide invaluable data on the AIDS epidemic which is collected by the CDC.

In the mid-seventies, hepatitis B became the "gay" sexually-transmitted disease which most intrigued the government scientists. Newly "liberated" homosexuals were anxious to cooperate with the government in matters of "gay" health.

THE GAY "HEPATITIS COHORTS" THAT FORMED UNDER THE AUSPICES OF THE GOVERNMENT EVENTUALLY BECAME THE EPIDEMIOLOGIC "MODEL" FOR AIDS IN AMERICA.

Dr. Wolf Szmuness was the mastermind who planned the hepatitis B vaccine trials in gay men. He was professor of epidemiology at the Columbia University School of Public Health, and chief of epidemiology at the New York City Blood Center in Manhattan.

According to Allan Chase (*Magic Shots*, 1982), Szmuness was a newcomer to the American medical and research communities. He was born in 1919 in Poland, and trained in the Soviet Union. Szmuness was active in hepatitis research when he was expelled from Poland by the communist government in an anti-semitic purge in 1968. He joined the New York Blood Center in 1969.

In planning the hepatitis experiment it was necessary to enroll a group of people who were at high-risk for the disease. There were a number of "high-risk" possibilities: Drug addicts, mentally deficient people, Chinese-Americans, Alaskan Indians, gay men, and patients and medical staff of kidney dialysis centers. Szmuness wrote, in a 1979 report, that he decided to choose homosexuals in order to avoid "serious legal and logistical problems."

Szmuness made the scientific requirements for partici-
pation in the New York City hepatitis vaccine study very
specific. Only men under the age of 40 were permitted
to enter the study. They had to be either homosexual or
bisexual. Straight men were excluded.

In order to eliminate men who were at lower risk for
hepatitis, Szmuness would not allow gay men over the
age of 40, or gays who were monogamous. Only
homosexuals who were young, healthy, and promiscuous
were wanted for the experiment.

The men had to be willing to receive a series of three
vaccinations, and to donate blood ten times. They were
required to provide name, address, and telephone
number for contact.

The federal government took a keen interest in the
trials. The experimental hepatitis B vaccine trials were
largely supported by grants from government agencies
such as the CDC, the NIH, and the National Institute
of Allergy and Infectious Diseases.

After screening the blood of almost ten thousand men,
a final group of 1083 were selected to participate in the
first Hepatitis B Vaccine Study. The experiment took
place at the New York City Blood Center in Manhattan,
during November 1978.

Characteristics of the gay men who were selected for
the final experiment included the following:

> the average age was 29
> the men were healthy
> more than half had NO history of venereal disease
> most were white and college educated

The vials containing the experimental hepatitis vaccine were produced and sealed in a government-supervised laboratory. As standard procedure, the vials would be unmarked except for an identifying number.

The experiment was "double-blinded." Neither the men nor the medical staff supervising the injections would know which vials contained the vaccine and which ones contained the placebo. The contents of the bottles could not be analysed.

The vials were coded. Only a few people who controlled the experiment knew the secrets of the code. And the experiment would not be decoded until the last gay man in the experiment was injected.

The biologic experiment was undertaken with the firm conviction that no one would be seriously harmed. The doctors had to be assured that there were no harmful substances in the vials that would be injurious to the men.

Everything in the experiment had to conform to the highest standards of medical science and excellence. Human errors could prove fatal.

The vaccine experiment was a dangerous game, and this one particularly so. The men in the experiment who would receive the three injections were from a segment of society that was the most hated and despised group in America.

When the young, healthy homosexual men lined up for their experimental injections, their faith and trust in the medical profession was implicit.

In November 1978, the first gay man was inoculated at the New York City Blood Center. By October 1979,

all the men in Szmuness' study were inoculated.
WITHIN A DECADE, MOST OF THE MEN IN
THE EXPERIMENT WOULD BE DOOMED TO DIE
OF AIDS.

Doctors in Manhattan first began to recognize cases
of "gay" cancer in young homosexual men in Manhattan
in 1979. As the number of cases mounted, the astute
physicians were convinced they were seeing a new and
fatal disease.

By 1979, government epidemiologists at the CDC had
finished a preliminary investigation of 4000 young gay
men, *in preparation for additional experimental hepatitis
B vaccine trials to be held in five more American cities.*
The names and addresses of the gays were garnered
from government VD clinics which functioned as health
care facilities for homosexuals. The epidemiologic
procedures were standard. Blood specimens were taken,
and answers to detailed questionnaires on homosexuality
were required from the men under surveillance.
This large epidemiologic study was undertaken at the
following VD clinics:

The Howard Brown Memorial Clinic in Chicago
The Gay Community Services Center in Los
Angeles
The San Francisco City Clinic
The Denver Metro Health Clinic
The St. Louis Sexually Transmitted Disease Center

The CDC study ended in July 1979. Over 60% of the

men had blood "markers" for hepatitis. San Francisco men had the highest blood marker rate (75%); St. Louis the lowest (50%).

The epidemiologists warned the gay community that anal-genital homosexual activity correlated most strongly with positive hepatitis blood tests.

These preliminary hepatitis B studies paved the way for the *second* series of experimental vaccine trials in five more American cities.

THE SECOND HEPATITIS B STUDY GROUP INCLUDED 1402 GAY MEN RECRUITED FROM GAY VD CLINICS IN SAN FRANCISCO, LOS ANGELES, DENVER, ST. LOUIS, AND CHICAGO. The group was similar to the New York City group in that the average age was 29. The men were healthy, and most were white (89%), and well educated.

The five-city hepatitis B experiments were supervised by a group of physicians headed by Donald Francis, an epidemiologist from the CDC. During the 1970s, Francis worked in Max Essex's animal cancer research lab at Harvard, trying to prove that feline leukemia virus was the cause of leukemia and lymphoma in cats. In 1984, Francis' ex-boss, Max Essex, co-discovered the AIDS virus with Robert Gallo.

THE EXPERIMENTAL VACCINE TRIALS IN THESE FIVE AMERICAN CITIES BEGAN IN MARCH 1980 (approximately one and a half years after the New York City trials ended). THE TRIALS CONTINUED UNTIL OCTOBER 1981.

The first diagnosed case of AIDS in a gay man from San Francisco appeared in the fall of 1980.

Within six months, the AIDS epidemic became "official."

Physicians could not understand why a mysterious infectious agent was killing young, previously healthy homosexual men.

The cause of the new disease was unknown, but many scientists were privately calling it the "gay plague."

References:

Shilts R: *The Mayor of Castro Street: The Life and Times of Harvey Milk,* St. Martin's Press, 1982.

Schreeder MT, Thompson SE, Hadler SC, et al: Hepatitis B in homosexual men: Prevalence of infection and factors related to transmission. J Infect Dis 146: 7-15, 1982.

Jaffe HW, Darrow WW, Echenberg DF, et al: The acquired immunodeficiency syndrome in a cohort of homosexual men. Ann Int Med 103: 210-214, 1985.

Szmuness W: Large scale efficacy trials of hepatitis B vaccines in the USA: Baseline data and protocols. J Med Virol 4: 327-340, 1979.

Chase A: *Magic Shots,* William Morrow and Company, New York, 1982, p335.

Szmuness W, Stevens CE, Harley EJ, et al: Hepatitis B vaccine: Demonstration of efficacy in a controlled clinical trial in a high-risk population. New Engl J Med 303: 833-841, 1980.

Francis DP, Hadler SC, Thompson SE, et al: The prevention of hepatitis B with vaccine. An Intern Med 97: 362-366, 1982.

CHAPTER SIX

The "Gay Plague"

The telltale signs of the gay plague were unmistakable. The most visible sign was the purple-red, cancerous skin tumors of Kaposi's sarcoma that grew and multiplied at an alarming rate on the bodies of the young gay men.

Doctors knew about this form of cancer for over a century. However, Kaposi's was an uncommon tumor, and physicians rarely saw patients with this disease. Before AIDS, this kind of cancer was almost never diagnosed in young American men.

It was quickly discovered that the dying gay men were markedly immunodeficient. For some unknown reason, their immune systems were being targeted for destruction. As a result, the men became highly susceptible to opportunistic infections.

The most common and serious opportunistic infection was a parasitic disease which caused a frequently fatal pneumonia, known as *Pneumocystis carinii* pneumonia. For some men, a dry cough and increasing shortness of breath could mean death from pneumocystis pneumonia within a few days. Other men might recover from the first pneumocystis infection, only to be stricken again and again. With rare exceptions, most AIDS patients diagnosed with pneumocystis pneumonia were dead within a year or two, at the most.

The immunodeficient men were constantly plagued

with all sorts of other opportunistic infections caused by viruses, bacteria, fungi, yeasts and parasites.

By 1981, the CDC defined AIDS as a primarily gay disease manifested by Kaposi's sarcoma, *Pneumocystis carinii* pneumonia, or both. These two major diseases (along with certain specified opportunistic infections) became the hallmarks for the diagnosis of AIDS.

The experts were convinced AIDS was a "new" disease, but I still had my doubts. It was true that gay men were dying of Kaposi's sarcoma, Pneumocystis pneumonia, and opportunistic infections. But none of these diseases were "new."

Kaposi's sarcoma was an "old" form of cancer, and was commonly found in blacks in central Africa. Pneumocystis pneumonia was known for a half century. Epidemics of pneumocystis had killed thousands of newborn babies and infants in central Europe during the 1930s, 40s, and 50s. In the 1960s and 1970s, cancer patients (especially children) were prone to develop *Pneumocystis carinii* pneumonia as a complication of chemotherapy.

Why were scientists calling AIDS a "new" disease? To me, AIDS was more like two "old" diseases that had suddenly become more common.

When AIDS became official in June 1981, the CDC was entrusted to see that the new disease would not become a serious problem in the United States. The agency assured "straight" America that there was little to worry about. After all, it *was* a "gay" disease.

The epidemiologists at the CDC were confident. The AIDS agent was most likely a new virus, and they had prepared for a possible epidemic of cancer at the

Biohazard Conference at Asilomar in 1973. At the meeting the virologists and epidemiologists had made careful provisions to track down a virus if one escaped from their cancer laboratories.

Now that the mysterious AIDS agent was "out" and the surveillance systems were in place, the government scientists would be able to monitor the spread of the new infectious disease into the gay community.

IN JANUARY 1979, TWO MONTHS AFTER THE BEGINNING OF THE NEW YORK CITY HEPATITIS VACCINE TRIALS, THE FIRST CASE OF AIDS WAS DISCOVERED IN A YOUNG GAY MAN LIVING IN NEW YORK CITY. THE WESTERN VACCINE TRIALS BEGAN IN MARCH 1980 IN L.A. AND SAN FRANCISCO. SEVEN MONTHS LATER, THE FIRST CASES OF AIDS WERE DISCOVERED IN THOSE CITIES.

A CDC report in August 1981, contained the following data on the first 26 cases:

All the cases were gay men
20 were from New York City
6 were from Los Angeles and San Francisco
25 were white; 1 was black
The average age was 39
Most were well educated

By the summer of 1982, AIDS was already accounting for 2-3% of all deaths in men between the ages of 25 and 45, living in New York, L.A. and San Francisco.

A new epidemic was born in the gay ghettos of Greenwich Village, West Hollywood, and in the homosexual districts of San Francisco. The mysterious disease was an unprecedented phenomenon for scientists. Never before had the epidemiologic experts at the CDC observed a "community-acquired" immunologic disease. There was no biological explanation for the event. The infectious disease experts could only surmise that a new infectious agent of unknown origin had been "introduced" into the gay community.

IN THE ABSENCE OF ANY KNOWN ETIOLOGIC AGENT, THE EXPERTS DECLARED THAT THE CAUSE OF THE EPIDEMIC WAS THE PROMISCUOUS HOMOSEXUAL LIFESTYLE — AN IMMORAL AND UNHEALTHY LIFESTYLE CHARACTERIZED BY THE USE AND ABUSE OF RECREATIONAL DRUGS AND ANAL SEX.

Was Strecker correct in his gut feeling that the AIDS virus was introduced into gays with the hepatitis B experimental vaccine? There did seem to be circumstantial evidence to suggest this possibility.

The most suggestive evidence was the striking epidemiologic profile of the gay men who had volunteered as guinea-pigs for the experimental hepatitis vaccine injections. THE EPIDEMIOLOGIC PROFILE OF THE GAY MEN WAS BASICALLY IDENTICAL TO THE PROFILE OF THE FIRST AIDS CASES THAT WERE REPORTED TO THE CDC.

The New York City Blood Center profile of the hepatitis B volunteers consisted of the following:

All the men were gay or bisexual
All were young and previously healthy
All were promiscuous
Most were well educated
Almost all were white

Was this just another epidemiologic coincidence? Or was there a tie-in between the hepatitis injections and the outbreak of the "gay plague" in those three large cities?

Strecker wasn't alone in suspecting a connection. According to a review of .the medical literature, a few other physicians and scientists had also considered the possibility.

To quell the concern about the safety of the hepatitis B vaccine, the CDC issued a report on the matter in September 1982. The federal agency claimed that NO cases of AIDS had developed in any hepatitis trial participant during a two-year followup period.

In a second report issued a year later, the CDC admitted that two homosexual men who had been vaccinated in the trials had come down with AIDS. However, the CDC again claimed that the outbreak of AIDS had no connection with the hepatitis trials in gays. As proof, the agency undertook a statistical analysis comparing the number of AIDS cases in the original cohort with other gays who were screened for the trials BUT WHO HAD NOT BEEN INJECTED WITH THE EXPERIMENTAL VACCINE. The CDC claimed there was NO statistical difference in AIDS cases between the two groups.

Early in the epidemic the government scientists

dismissed any connection between the hepatitis vaccine trials in gays and the outbreak of AIDS in gay people. However, the AIDS experts were busy establishing other epidemiologic "connections" to gay men in Manhattan.

After the "official" onset of the "gay plague" in 1981, the surveillance of homosexuals by United States Public Health officials intensified. By 1982, the surveillance system of gays had also been transformed into an overseas operation.

In December 1981, three years after the first New York City AIDS cases were reported to the CDC, an epidemiological study of a cohort of gay men in Denmark was undertaken. At this early stage of the epidemic, it was obvious that certain U.S. and Danish scientists already suspected a "Danish connection" to AIDS.

The Danish study began urgently after four gay Danes were diagnosed with AIDS in 1981. ALL FOUR DANES HAD SEXUAL CONTACT WITH HOMO-SEXUAL MEN IN THE U.S.A., OR WITH AMERI-CANS TRAVELING IN DENMARK OR ELSEWHERE IN EUROPE.

The study was arranged and supported by the National Cancer Institute (NCI), the National Institute of Health (NIH), and the Danish Cancer Society. Robert Biggar,a physician-epidemiologist from the NIH, was the chief American investigator in the study.

The Danish researchers were convinced a contagious agent was involved in AIDS, and they were sure the agent was brought to Denmark via American gay men.

As in America, the Danish investigators solicited

volunteers through homosexual organizations. They chose men from Copenhagen and the small town of Aarthus. The purpose of the study was to determine the mens' sexual lifestyle and "virus exposure."

The 259 selected gay Danes were carefully questioned about sexual contacts with American men, especially during the years 1980-1981, either in Denmark or during travel abroad. As usual, blood was taken and stored for virus and immune system testing.

The blood test results of the study rapidly refuted the prevailing belief (in 1982) that the cytomegalovirus (CMV) might be the cause of AIDS. By 1983, most sophisticated government AIDS researchers had already eliminated CMV as the cause of AIDS. The top AIDS investigators were busy hunting for a "new" virus.

The most important revelations of the Danish study were published in 1984, after Robert Gallo tested the stored (1982) Danish blood samples for AIDS virus antibodies. Remarkably, 22 (9%) of the 259 Danes had AIDS antibodies in their blood samples collected in 1982. MOST OF THESE MEN HAD TRAVELED TO THE U.S.A. DURING THE YEARS 1980-1981! Fourteen of 19 antibody-positive Danes had sex with American men during the year 1980, or had sexual exposure to a European man with AIDS.

It was obvious the AIDS virus had been "introduced" into Denmark through sexual contact between Danish men and gay men from high-risk areas.

Another report on the Danish study published in *JAMA* in March 1984, stressed the highly damaging immune effects of the AIDS virus. DANES WHO WENT TO AMERICA IN 1980-1981 WERE ALMOST

EIGHT TIMES AS LIKELY TO BE IMMUNODE-
PRESSED WHEN COMPARED TO THOSE WHO
DIDN'T.

Although Danish gays proved to be less promiscuous
than their American counterparts, it mattered little. The
Danish study indicated that promiscuity was not a
requirement for AIDS. All that was necessary was the
unfortunate choice of an infected American gay man as
a sex partner after the year 1978 — the year the
hepatitis experiments began.

By 1982, top government epidemiologists also clearly
realized that New York City was a high-risk area for
AIDS. In the spring of that year, Biggar and a group of
researchers from the NCI were already busy investigating
the spread of AIDS from New York City into Washington, D.C.

Biggar's group settled into the medical offices of two
Washington physicians whose clientele was "90% likely
to be gay or bisexual." A companion study was also
undertaken in the offices of two New York City doctors
"with a similar patient population."

Their report, issued in 1985, showed IMMUNE
SYSTEM ABNORMALITIES IN THE WASHINGTON
GAY MEN WHO HAD SEX WITH NEW YORK
CITY GAYS. The epidemiologists issued a grave
warning: "There are currently few, if any, large
American cities where promiscuous and anonymous
homosexual activity can safely be considered free from
the risk of AIDS."

Although government researchers proved how quickly
the infectious agent of AIDS could spread from city-to-
city and from continent-to-continent, the U.S. govern-

ment showed no concern about protecting the public from AIDS. Only a few, carefully-selected government scientists were funded to track the spread of the new and deadly virus that zeroed in on young and healthy homosexuals. Over and over again, the American public was reassured that AIDS was a "gay" disease resulting from a promiscuous and licentious lifestyle.

Although government scientists carefully avoided mention of any "connection" between the experimental hepatitis vaccine trials and the outbreak of AIDS in the gay community, the possible "connection" was occasionally raised in the medical literature.

As late as October 1983, several infectious disease specialists reported that AIDS might be related to the hepatitis vaccine. A hepatitis connection was suspected because 93% OF THEIR AIDS PATIENTS TESTED POSITIVE FOR HEPATITIS B BLOOD MARKERS. Because the hepatitis B vaccine was manufactured from the blood of gays who carried the hepatitis virus, the physicians feared "the AIDS agent could also be included in the vaccine." Predictably, the CDC again reassured them the hepatitis vaccine was safe.

The safety of the hepatitis vaccine was also defended by Cladd Stevens, who collaborated with Wolf Szmuness in the New York City experimental trials in gays. When Szmuness died of cancer in 1982, Stevens became the official spokesperson for the vaccine trials. In a May 1983 report, she readily admitted that one gay man had been diagnosed with AIDS in November 1982, four years after receiving the vaccine. A second gay man developed AIDS two years after the vaccine injections.

But like the CDC, Stevens provided statistics to prove that 16 AIDS cases were diagnosed in a group of 3646 gay men who had been screened for the trials BUT WHO DID NOT PARTICIPATE IN THE EXPERIMENT.

According to Stevens, "No cases have occurred in vaccine recipients from populations at low-risk for AIDS, and THERE IS NO EXCESS INCIDENCE IN THE HIGH-RISK POPULATION. I am already aware of several cases of hepatitis B among people who refused to take the vaccine for fear of acquiring AIDS. This potential tragedy is preventable. Those of us at risk should not hestitate to take the vaccine and recommend it to others."

(In 1983, the year Stevens penned this report, ONE OF EVERY THREE MEN EXPERIMENTALLY INJECTED UNDER HER SUPERVISION WERE ALREADY INFECTED WITH THE AIDS VIRUS. In 1986, Stevens and her colleagues would officially report statistics suggesting that the MAJORITY of the gay men who received the experimental vaccine at the New York City Blood Center were infected with the AIDS virus. In this shocking report, Stevens did not cite her May 1983 previous report disclaiming "no excess [AIDS] incidence in the high-risk population.")

Prior to the discovery of the AIDS virus in 1984, the CDC and the vaccine experimenters repeatedly assured the public that the commercial hepatitis B vaccine was safe. However, Abbott Laboratories, which manufactures the vaccine, was cautious in this regard. In a commercial brochure urging gay men to take the vaccine, Abbott explained the AIDS risk in this statement:

"Many people are concerned about the possible transmission of AIDS and Kaposi's sarcoma; it is unknown whether these are conveyed by blood or blood products. The current hepatitis B vaccine, although produced from the pooled blood of chronic (virus) carriers, is manufactured utilizing several processes believed to inactivate all known groups of viruses."

Was it a coincidence that AIDS broke out in New York City shortly after the trials? And was it another coincidence that AIDS began in the west coast cities of L.A. and San Francisco ONE YEAR AFTER the disease appeared in New York? Or did the one-year lag time on the west coast have something to do with the fact that the western hepatitis trials occurred one year behind the New York City trials?

Although the CDC wasn't concerned about the vaccine's safety, the public was. The reason was natural. Gay men were coming down with AIDS, and the commercial hepatitis B vaccine was made from "pooled" blood donated by gay men who were hepatitis B virus carriers. In July 1982, at the time the commercial vaccine was released for public use, nobody knew for sure what was causing AIDS. As a result, people were afraid to take the vaccine.

AIDS experts like Marcus Conant, co-director of the Kaposi's sarcoma clinic in San Francisco, was also wary of the new vaccine. He wrote: "An interesting speculation is the association between hepatitis B and the new AIDS syndrome. Of the 50 patients with Kaposi's sarcoma whom we have evaluated in San Francisco, 90% have been seropositive for hepatitis B. Could it be that the new AIDS agent is an incomplete viral particle which requires for its replication certain helper functions from the hepatitis B virus?"

The commercial hepatitis vaccine bombed badly for good reasons. In the mind of the public, the vaccine was associated with "gay" blood, "gay" hepatitis, and "gay" AIDS.

In 1984, after the new AIDS virus was accepted as the "sole" cause of AIDS, the tenuous link between "gay" AIDS and the experimental vaccine trials in gay men was dropped completely.

Nevertheless, as late as 1985, James Curran of the CDC continued to reassure physicians about the safety of the *commercial* hepatitis vaccine by claiming that "epidemiologic studies have not detected an association between the vaccine and AIDS in cases of AIDS reported to the CDC, and in members of AIDS risk groups who received hepatitis B vaccine."

In 1986, Cladd Stevens, *et al* did a second followup study of 212 gay men in New York City who were injected three times with the original experimental hepatitis B vaccine during the period November 1978 and October 1979. Like the Danish study, the purpose of Stevens' study was to determine the homosexual activity of the cohort, and to determine the spread of the AIDS virus "into" the group during the years 1979-1984.

Men in the original group who had been injected with the experimental vaccine and who later came down with AIDS were excluded from the study. Stevens gave no reason why she excluded the men with AIDS, nor did she state the actual number of men from the original group who were rejected because they developed AIDS.

The spread of the AIDS virus among the men was determined by checking AIDS antibodies in the "old" (1978-1979) blood samples collected from the 212 gay volunteers during the first year of the hepatitis study. In addition, the researchers checked for AIDS antibodies in later blood samples which had been collected from the men every 3-6 months until the year 1984.

AMAZINGLY, 6.6% OF THE ORIGINAL GROUP OF 212 MEN WHO HAD BEEN INJECTED WITH THE VACCINE HAD AIDS VIRUS ANTIBODIES IN THEIR BLOOD SAMPLES COLLECTED DUR-ING NOVEMBER 1978 AND OCTOBER 1979! This was additional proof that the AIDS virus was "intro-duced" into the New York City gay community TWO YEARS BEFORE THE "OFFICIAL" BEGINNING OF THE AIDS EPIDEMIC IN 1981!

By 1981, over 20% of the original 212 men had a positive virus antibody test; by 1984 (the end of Stevens' study period) over 40% tested positive. Most of these "positive" men were immunodeficient.

On the basis of Stevens' projected (post-1984) statistics, it is likely that the vast majority of the men who volunteered for the experimental hepatitis B vaccine trial now have AIDS virus antibodies. ACCORDING TO THE AIDS EXPERTS, AS MANY AS 50% (AND POSSIBLY AS MANY AS 100%) OF THESE ANTI-BODY-POSITIVE GAY MEN WILL DIE OF AIDS OR AIDS-RELATED DISEASES IN THE FUTURE.

Stevens' gloomy statistics and prognosis for men in the original hepatitis study group were overlooked in an interview with Lawrence Altman of *The New York*

Times (AIDS mystery: Why do some infected men stay healthy?, June 30, 1987). Instead, her comments were upbeat on the matter. She remarked about 13 men in the original group who were "already infected with the AIDS virus and had lived nine years without developing AIDS." Stevens was "astonished" that all 13 men had "perfectly normal" immune systems. "More astonishing" was her claim that "for unknown reasons only one of the 87 people in the New York City Blood Center study who were found to have become infected with the AIDS virus since 1981 has developed AIDS."

No mention was made to Altman of the fate of the additional 1000 men who volunteered for the original New York City study, nor did she mention her previously published 1986 report which implied that almost one-half of those men were infected with the AIDS virus. (For reasons best known to the CDC, the total number of AIDS deaths in the gay men who volunteered for the six original hepatitis cohorts has never appeared anywhere in the scientific literature).

I was amazed to learn in Altman's article that the CDC has agreed to finance future research inquiring into the fate of gay men who volunteered for the experimental trials in Chicago and Denver. Such studies "are planned to examine and test for AIDS virus infection in all the subjects who can be found, with their permission. The research in San Francisco is being expanded to include all the regional participants, not just the small sample already selected, for more extensive study."

In 1987, a new "recombinant" hepatitis B vaccine

(Recombivax-HB) was released to the public. The new vaccine was manufactured in "yeasts" by recombinant DNA technology.

In a *JAMA* editorial (May 15, 1987) praising the development of the new vaccine, F. Blaine Hollinger cited previous scientific studies which purportedly proved the original *experimental* hepatitis B vaccine was safe. He complained about "the unfounded fear" and "misguided concern" of acquiring AIDS from the *commercial* vaccine. Although Hollinger cited six of Stevens' previous reports as proof of the vaccine's safety, no mention was made of her 1986 *JAMA* paper which showed that over 40% of the injected men in the New York City experimental vaccine trials were infected with the AIDS virus as early as 1984.

The published reports of hepatitis experts like Stevens and Hollinger serve as evidence to prove that the vaccine experiments on gay people had nothing to do with the AIDS outbreak in the gay community. Allusions of any connection would, no doubt, be considered coincidental by these scientists.

But in truth, the scientific "evidence" provided by "statistics" proves the old adage that WITH THE PROPER STATISTICS YOU CAN PROVE ANYTHING.

With the discovery of the AIDS virus in 1984, and the subsequent development of a blood test for AIDS virus antibodies, the virologists had their final proof that AIDS was a "new" disease caused by a "new" virus.

There was no proof the virus caused Kaposi's sarcoma, but that didn't seem to bother the AIDS experts. No scientist of stature questioned the new government dictum that the AIDS virus was the "sole" cause of AIDS.

Through AIDS antibody blood testing of pre-1978 stored blood, the scientists proved that THE NEW AIDS VIRUS DID NOT EXIST IN AMERICA BEFORE 1978.

In the face of this overwhelming evidence, I finally had to admit to myself that there was more to the AIDS epidemic than just the presence of cancer bacteria. The AIDS virus was new and frightening. It had the capacity to destroy the immune system, and to *unleash* cancer, pneumocystis pneumonia, and opportunistic infections. According to the CDC, "old" diseases like Kaposi's and pneumocystis pneumonia were now synonymous with AIDS — at least in gays and other "high-risk" people.

There was something fishy about this new kind of AIDS science. Nobody wanted to examine the holes in the theories that were quickly disseminated to the media. Conflicting scientific information was quickly swept under the carpet. I wondered why. It took me a long time to figure it out.

There was complete agreement that the AIDS virus had been "introduced" into the United States through the male homosexual population in Manhattan, sometime around the years 1978-1979. The negative testing of old (pre-1978) blood for AIDS virus antibodies had supplied that proof.

Early in the epidemic, scientists were unable to explain how the AIDS virus was "introduced" into large numbers of gay men residing primarily in three American cities (New York, San Francisco and Los Angeles). However, with the discovery of the AIDS virus in 1984, certain AIDS experts (primarily virologists and immunologists) had already composed several theories which attempted to explain how the AIDS virus was seeded into American gay males.

The scientific theories include:

1. The AIDS virus originated in the African "green" monkey. The virus "jumped" species, and spread (through monkey or insect bites, the ingestion of contaminated meat, or bestiality?) into the human heterosexual population of Central Africa. The virus then spread to Haiti, and eventually to Manhattan.

2. The African AIDS virus spread to Haiti through heterosexual contact between central Africans and Haitians.

3. The AIDS virus was "picked up" in Haiti by vacationing gays from Manhattan as a result of homosexual activities with Haitian men. These gay New Yorkers brought AIDS to America.

4. The AIDS virus may have spread in Haiti through animal blood-letting ceremonies during voodoo rituals.

All these theories are now widely accepted by doctors and scientists, and the theories are rarely questioned.

But there is one theory that is never mentioned in conventional scientific circles. And that is the theory promoted by Strecker and a few others.

According to Strecker's theory:

1 The AIDS virus is a "man-made" virus which was

engineered in a cancer-virus laboratory.

2. This man-made AIDS virus was deliberately (or perhaps accidentally) "introduced" into humans by way of injections during vaccination programs involving American gay men, black Africans, and Haitians.

As my inquiry into the origin of AIDS progressed, Strecker's theories seemed more plausable than the explanations supplied by the government.

He kept saying, "If you read and you think, it's the most logical conclusion you can come to as a scientist."

There was no absolute proof that the hepatitis B vaccine trials were the key to the origin of AIDS in American gays, but there were so many clues and coincidences, and such obvious connections between the cancer researchers and AIDS, that I was surprised no one but Strecker had ever hit upon them.

It also became very clear that it was impossible to unravel the origin of AIDS and the AIDS virus without knowledge of the politics of cancer, the politics of the medical establishment, and the politics of AIDS.

One thing I had learned in my twenty-five years as a scientific researcher was that you didn't discount the opinions of other scientific investigators until you checked out all the facts. Strecker was correct. There was a hepatitis — AIDS connection. What you wanted to make of it depended on how much you trusted medical science.

I was surprised to learn that much of the scientific knowledge that had accumulated on the "spread" of AIDS in America has come from the continuing surveillance and blood testing of large groups of gay and bisexual men, dating back to the original hepatitis B vaccine trials during the years 1978-1981.

Was it coincidental that those were the beginning years of the AIDS epidemic, and the years just before AIDS became "official?"

Strecker always seemed to have interesting answers to my questions about the AIDS connection to the hepatitis trials in gays.

I asked him about the other cities involved in the trials. Was there foul play in Chicago, St. Louis and Denver?

Strecker wasn't sure. "It could be that the AIDS virus was introduced only in New York City, L.A., and San Francisco. Or *another* virus could have been seeded into the other three cities. Or those three other cities could have served as *controls* for the experiment."

What about the incubation period of the AIDS virus? Remembering that the discovery of the first New York City AIDS case coincided closely with the initiation of the trials, I asked Strecker whether such a short incubation period would have been possible.

He responded, "The incubation period of the virus would depend on the dosage of the virus. If you injected a *heavy* dose directly into the body, the incubation period might be very, very short."

Strecker also considered the strong possibility that *only some (or perhaps only a few)* of the men in the trials might have been injected with the AIDS virus. In any case, the incubation period in someone who received a *heavy infection dose* of virus would be shorter than the incubation period of the same virus that was picked up "naturally" in a sexual encounter.

I believed very strongly that in order to pinpoint the initial "introduction" of the AIDS virus into gay men, IT WAS ESSENTIAL TO STUDY CAREFULLY THE EPIDEMIOLOGAL PROFILE OF THE VERY EAR-LIEST CASES. As the Danish and the Washington-New York epidemiological studies indicated, the virus spread rapidly from person-to-person, and from city-to-city, and from continent-to-continent. THE EXACT POINT OF AIDS VIRUS INTRODUCTION WOULD BE RAPIDLY OBSCURED UNLESS ONE STUDIED ONLY THE EARLIEST CASES.

To Strecker, the origin of AIDS was elementary. The AIDS virus was "put into" the gay community, most probably during the vaccine trials.

Ironically, Strecker's simplistic answers to the origin of the AIDS virus in the gay community sounded a bit like those of Robert Gallo, who discovered the AIDS virus.

In an interview with James D'Eramo (*New York Native*, August 24, 1984), Gallo was asked why gay men were the first victims of the AIDS virus. Gallo answered, "They are homosexuals because they were the ones exposed. Forget all the other hocus-pocus. Why them? No one knows. . . it was acquired."

Gallo was adamant about the AIDS virus being the "sole" cause of the disease. Like Strecker, he believed the "dose" of the virus was important in determining its infectivity.

He told D'Eramo: "If I tell you you're going to be a test experiment, and I inoculate you intravenously with a walloping amount of the virus, you're going to get the disease."

After all my reading, I was convinced that there was a tie-in between the hepatitis vaccine trials and the AIDS outbreak. There were too many peculiar "coincidences" and "connections" between the cancer and the AIDS establishment. And behind this powerful force was the additional might of the U.S. government.

Was is it just another "coincidence" that the New York Blood Center in Manhattan was located at the epicenter of the "new" epidemic. And still another "coincidence" that the plague in gays started in Manhattan shortly after the experimental trials at the Blood Center? And a "coincidence" that the gay hepatitis cohorts became the "model" for the spread of the AIDS epidemic in America?

Who was Wolf Szmuness, the mastermind behind the vaccine trials? Why was a recent (1969) immigrant to America chosen to head one of the most important medical experiments of this century? Why was he picked by the U.S. government over all other American-trained epidemiologists? Why would the government turn over millions of dollars in research grants to a foreign doctor schooled in the Soviet Union?

How could Szmuness attain a full Professorship at Columbia University within a few short years? Why was he chosen as Chief of Epidemiology at the Blood Center? As an exile from Poland, what were his brilliant professional credentials which allowed him to head a dangerous human experiment involving thousands of American gay men?

Late in my investigation, I uncovered a medical paper

in an obscure medical journal that contained a brief sketch of his life, and answered some of these questions. The posthumous mini-biography (Reflections on Wolf Szmuness, published in *Proceedings in Clinical and Biologic Research*, Volume 182, 1985, pages 3-10) was written by a colleague, Aaron Kellner, who is associated with the New York Blood Center.

Szmuness, a Jew born in Poland in 1919, was a young medical student in Lublin in eastern Poland when the Nazis attacked that country in the summer of 1939. When Poland was quickly partitioned by Germany and Russia, Szmuness was sent to Siberia as a prisoner. His family in western Poland were all murdered by the Nazis in the Holocaust. Szmuness' years in exile in Siberia were "a long, dark period that he was most reluctant to talk about."

After release from detention in 1946 he was somehow allowed to finish his medical education in Tomsk in central Russia. While a student, he married a Russian woman. He specialized in epidemiology, and when his wife contracted a nearly fatal case of hepatitis, Szmuness decided that the study of that disease would be his life's work.

In 1959, the Soviets allowed him and his family to return to Poland "where he held a series of minor positions as an epidemiologist in municipal and regional health departments."

During this time, he told Kellner "an interesting story." Due to exhaustion and stress from work, he applied to the authorities for a vacation at a rest home. Szmuness was allowed to share a room with a Catholic priest. A remarkable friendship developed and the two men corresponded "for a long time thereafter." The Polish priest eventually became the first Polish Pope in Catholic history: the current, anti-communist and anti-gay Pope John Paul II.

In 1969, in another strange twist of fate, the communists allowed Szmuness and his wife and daughter to attend a scientific meeting in Italy. While there, he and his family defected to the West. (Kellner's account is at odds with Allan Chase's story [*Magic Shots*, page 333] that Szmuness came to America because "the Polish government in 1968 suddenly started to drive those of its few Jews who had survived the Holocaust out of Poland.")

He arrived in Manhattan with $15 in his pocket. Through the intervention of Walsh McDermott, Professor of Public Health at New York Hospital - Cornell Medical Center, Szmuness miraculously secured a position as a "lab tech" at the New York City Blood Center.

Within a few years, Szmuness was given his own lab, and a separate department of epidemiology at the Center was created for him. "In what must be record time, he was leap-frogged to full Professorship at the Columbia School of Public Health."

By the mid-70s, he was a world authority on hepatitis and "transfusion medicine." In another unbelievable occurrence, he was invited back to Moscow in 1975 to give a scientific presentation. As a defector he was terrified to set foot in the Soviet Union, but his colleagues assured him he would have the full protection of the State Department. He finally agreed to go, and his return to Russia was a scientific triumph.

By the late 1970s he had been awarded millions of dollars in grant money and was "phenomenally successful" in his hepatitis work which had tremendous "global implications." Szmuness' meteoric and unprecedented rise to world prominence was halted by his death from cancer in 1982. (A 1983 paper published after his death detailed a new experimental hepatitis B vaccine program in Kangwane that would use black South African infants as experimental subjects.)

As a defector, could Szmuness have been a Russian agent? Or could he have been playing both sides of the field by working as a "double-agent" for America and the Soviet Union? His life story was proof that he was honored by both countries. Although the scientific world would undoubtedly laugh at these questions, Szmuness' professional life in the communist and the free-world was filled with the oddest of circumstances and coincidences.

As a precaution against escape, it is my understanding that potential defectors from communist countries are *never* allowed the opportunity to travel outside the country with their entire family. Yet, Szmuness defected with his family in tow. After defecting, how was it possible to arrange his safe return to Russia "to present a scientific paper." Undoubtedly, cooperation at the highest levels of *both* governments was necessary to accomplish this feat.

A review of Szmuness' published research projects during the 1970s clearly shows intimate connections between the Blood Center and the NIH, the NCI, the FDA, the WHO, and the Cornell, Yale, and Harvard Schools of Public Health. In addition, a 1980 paper reveals close ties with the Moscow Ministry of Health

and the Russian Academy of Medical Science. Szmuness'
other global connections included the International
Agency for Research on Cancer (IARC) in Lyons,
France, and close ties to third-world African countries.
In a 1973 research project, the services of the Sengalese
Army were employed to secure blood specimens in one
of Szmuness' many African ventures.

In evaluating Szmuness and the role the hepatitis
experiment might have had in unleashing the AIDS
epidemic, the close U.S. and Soviet scientific ties should
not be overlooked. It must be borne in mind that
America and the Soviet Union have one thing very
much in common. AT THE TOP LEVEL OF GOV-
ERNMENT, BOTH NATIONS ARE WHITE RACIST
SOCIETIES. AIDS has the potential to wipe out large
masses of non-white, third-world people, especially in
black Africa. This future holocaust will drastically alter
the global political and economic structure. These
forthcoming changes and upheavals could prove extremely beneficial to *both* the United States and the
Soviet Union in their half-century struggle for world
power and domination.

In closing his story of Wolf Szmuness, Aaron Kellner
wrote: "He was the quintessential doctor's doctor. Most
physicians in their professional careers influence the lives
of a few hundred or a few thousand people. Some
fortunate ones can influence the lives of a few million. It
is the rare physician who, like Wolf Szmuness, is given
the grace to touch the lives of billions of people — those
living on this planet and generations yet unborn."

A decade after the epidemic, most American AIDS

experts still believed in the "green monkey" theory, as originally proposed by Robert Gallo when he "discovered" the AIDS virus in 1984. Ten years after AIDS, Gallo continues to be the most important and influential expert on the epidemic, and few establishment scientists dare to disagree with Gallo's story. Having rapidly convinced the scientists — the doctors, the media, and the public, all fell in line.

But people like Strecker were convinced there was foul play in Africa and Haiti, just like there had been foul play in New York, Los Angeles and San Francisco. With time, he was sure I would also discover the truth about Africa and Haiti.

Like the experts, I believed in the "connection" between American AIDS and Africa. After all, I was an expert on the subject of Kaposi's sarcoma. And Kaposi's was a common cancer in central Africa, and it was a common cancer in gays with AIDS. Only a fool would fail to recognize the African "connection" to AIDS.

But after I met Strecker, I began to study African AIDS more carefully and critically. With time, I became aware of a different kind of AIDS "connection" between the two continents.

The connection seemed to involve a whole lot more than just green monkeys.

References:

CDC: Kaposi's sarcoma and Pneumocystis pneumonia among homosexual men — New York City and California. MMWR 30: 305-308, 1981.

Levine AS: The epidemic of acquired immune dysfunction in homosexual men and its sequelae — opportunistic infections, Kaposi's sarcoma, and other malignancies: An update and interpretation. Cancer Treatment Reports 66: 1391-1395, 1982.

DeWys WD, Curran J, Henle W, et al: Workshop on Kaposi's sarcoma: Meeting report. Cancer Treatment Reports 66: 1387-1390, 1982.

CDC: Hepatitis B virus vaccine safety: Report of an inter-agency group. MMWR 31:465-467, 1982.

CDC: The safety of hepatitis B virus vaccine. MMWR 32: 134-136, 1983.

McDonald MI, Hamilton JD, Durack DT: Hepatitis B surface antigen could harbour the infective agent of AIDS. Lancet 2: 882-884, 1983.

Stevens CE: No increased incidence of AIDS in recipients of hepatitis B vaccine. New England Journal of Medicine 308: 11631165, 1983.

Curran JW, Morgan WM, Hardy AM, et al: The epidemiology of AIDS: Current status and future prospects. Science 229, 1352-1357, 1985.

Stevens CE, Taylor PE, Zang EA, et al: Human T-cell lymphotropic virus type III infection in a cohort of homosexual men in New York City. JAMA 255: 2167-2172, 1986.

Hollinger FB: Hepatitis B vaccines — to switch or not to switch. JAMA 257: 2634-2636, 1987.

Moss AR, Bacchetti P, Osmond D, et al: Incidence of the acquired immunodeficiency syndrome in San Francisco, 1980-1983. J Infect Dis 152:152-161, 1985.

Conant MA, Moss A, Dritz S, et al: Changing patterns of sexually-transmitted diseases over the past 15 years, in *AIDS: The Epidemic of Kaposi's Sarcoma and Opportunistic Infections.* Friedman-Kien AE, and Laubenstein LJ (Eds), Masson Publishing USA, New York, 1984, pp 263-278.

Gerstoft J, Malchow-Moller A, Bygbjerg I, et al: Severe acquired immunodeficiency in European homosexual men. Brit Med J 285: 17-19, 1982.

Melbye M, Biggar RJ, Ebbesen P, et al: Lifestyle and antibody studies among homosexual men in Denmark. Arch Pathol Microbiol Scand (Sect B) 91: 357-364, 1983.

Biggar RJ, Andersen HK, Ebbesen P, et al: Seminal fluid excretion of cytomegalovirus related to immunosuppression in homosexual men. Brit Med J 286: 210-212, 1983.

Melbye M, Biggar RJ, Ebbesen P, et al: Seroepidemiology of HTLV-III antibody in Danish homosexual men: Prevalence, transmission, and disease outcome. Brit Med

J 289: 573-575, 1984.

Biggar RJ, Melbye M, Ebesen P, et al: Low T-lymphocyte ratios in homosexual men: Epidemiologic evidence for a transmissible agent. JAMA 251: 1441-1446, 1984.

Goedert JJ, Biggar RJ, Winn DM, et al: Decreased helper T lymphocytes in homosexual men: Sexual contact in high-incidence areas for the acquired immunodeficiency syndrome. Amer J Epidemiol 121: 629-636, 1985.

Prozesky OW, Szmuness W, Stevens CE, et al: Baseline epidemiological studies for a hepatitis B vaccine trial in Kangwane. South African Med J 64: 891-893, 1983.

Holland P, Golosova T, Szmuness W, et al: Viral hepatitis markers in Soviet and American blood donors. Transfusion 20:504-510, 1980.

CHAPTER SEVEN

The African and Haitian Connection

When I first met Strecker that fateful day in August 1986, it was depressing to hear his prediction that the black population of Africa was doomed. The statement seemed so outrageous and unbelievably pessimistic. But six months later, *TIME* magazine (February 16, 1987) quoted Sam Okware, the Ugandan Minister of Health, as saying: "In the year 2000, one in every two sexually-active adults will be infected."

Along with this biological holocaust, Africans must contend with the belief of AIDS experts who agree unquestioningly that AIDS started in Africa. This belief pervades the science of AIDS in spite of clear-cut epidemiological evidence which indicates that AIDS STARTED IN NEW YORK CITY AROUND THE SAME TIME IT STARTED IN CENTRAL AFRICA, AND IN HAITI.

Gallo, (the co-discoverer of the AIDS virus), continues to promote his theory of an African origin for AIDS in articles like the one he wrote for *Scientific American* (The AIDS virus, January 1987). According to Gallo, "AIDS is probably the result of a new infection of human beings that began in central Africa, perhaps as recently as the 50s. From there it probably spread to the

111

Caribbean and then to the U.S. and Europe."

Gallo's view is supported by his friend and colleague, Max Essex of Harvard, also a co-discoverer of the AIDS virus. Essex was the first to find a virus related to the HTLV-3 (AIDS) virus in African green monkeys, and to suggest that the monkey virus "may well be an ancestor of the AIDS agent."

Not surprisingly, Essex named his new monkey virus "simian T-cell lymphotropic virus 3" (STLV-3). According to Gallo, "although STLV-3 is a closer relative of HTLV-3 than any other animal retrovirus, the relation between them is not close. Nor is the monkey virus pathogenic in its usual (monkey) host."

To complicate matters, American and French scientists have found additional "new" family members of HTLV viruses in West Africans. One of these new "human" viruses discovered by Essex, and named HTLV-4, is "remarkably similar" to Essex's new AIDS-like monkey virus.

Some scientists have privately disputed the identity of Essex's "new" HTLV-4 AIDS-like virus by declaring that the new human virus is actually a "contaminant" monkey virus that worked its way into Essex's cultures (much like HeLa cell contamination). In the future, more "new" African AIDS-like viruses will undoubtedly be discovered and will provoke continued controversy as to their authenticity.

Strecker believes the discovery of new African AIDS-like viruses is a natural outgrowth of biologic warfare experiments. According to his "Bioattack Alert" (March, 1986), the "plan" for Africa was clearly spelled out in a memoranda contained in the *Bulletin of the World*

Health Organization (Virus-associated immunopathology: animal models and implications for human disease. 1. Effects of viruses on the immune system, immune complex diseases, and antibody-mediated immunologic injury, Volume 47, pages 257-264, 1972).

The memoranda revealed that WHO scientists had a clear knowledge of virus-induced AIDS-like diseases years before the outbreak of the AIDS epidemic. Researchers were aware that infection with certain viruses, especially leukemia and lymphoma retroviruses, could result in *"selective damage"* to specific cells of the immune system, particularly white blood cells known as T and B-lymphocytes (the cells destroyed by the AIDS virus). Scientists also knew that "depression of the immune response might trigger or enhance the growth of certain (cancer) tumors."

The American, English, Dutch, Swiss, and Australian scientists who wrote the memoranda made three recommendations concerning these cancer-causing and immunosuppressive AIDS-like viruses.

First, "a systematic evaluation of the effects of viruses should be undertaken."

Second, the effects of virus infection on different white blood cell types, such as T and B-cells, should be studied.

Third, it should be ascertained whether certain viruses can "selectively" depress the immune system by affecting T-cell function as opposed to B-cell function.

In Part Two of the memoranda (*Bulletin WHO* 47:265-272), the WHO scientists further explained the specific immunodeficiences that could be produced in laboratory experimental animals inoculated with certain viruses. They stressed that these new findings had serious "implications for human disease and clinical research."

The WHO officials wrote that "while it would not be possible to conduct similar research on human subjects, the knowledge acquired in animal studies may be applicable in human disease. . . (and) the theoretical concepts and technical methods summarized in this memorandum may be usefully applied to the study of suspected immunopathological manifestations in human disease, including autoimmune reactions."

In the same year (1972) another official document published in the *Federation Proceedings* greatly intrigued Strecker. The report was obscurely titled "Biological significance of histocompatibility antigens," and contained a Committee report on a July 1970 "workshop" held at the National Institutes of Health (NIH) in Bethesda, Maryland. The workshop was jointly sponsored by the John E. Fogarty International Center for Advanced Study in the Health Sciences, and the World Health Organization.

A few quotes from this highly technical paper attest to the idea that scientists in the early 1970s already had a profound understanding of the immune system and the mechanisms of the T-cell immunologic response.

For example, the Committee wrote: "There are good grounds for believing that the relative strength (of the immune response) is largely a function of the relative numbers of unprimed T-cells which can recognize the (viral) antigens as being foreign. . . however, there is also now good evidence that the T- cells are not omnipotential. THE T-CELLS RESPONDING TO

ONE STRONG ANTIGEN CAN BE SELECTIVELY KILLED and the remaining cell population retains responsiveness to another antigen."

The Committee "visualized" a number of "useful experimental approaches" to determine the immune response in human beings. "ONE WOULD BE A STUDY OF THE RELATIONSHIP OF (GENETIC) HL-A TYPE TO THE IMMUNE RESPONSE, BOTH HUMORAL AND CELLULAR, TO WELL-DEFINED BACTERIAL AND VIRAL ANTIGENS DURING PREVENTIVE VACCINATION. THIS APPROACH WOULD BE PARTICULARLY INFORMATIVE WHEN APPLIED TO SIBSHIPS."

The word "sibships" undoubtedly refers to children of the same family. "During preventive vaccination" most likely means that children would be given "experimental" infectious agents (i.e. "bacterial and viral antigens") ALONG WITH "ROUTINE" (i.e "preventative") VACCINATIONS.

THE WHO OFFICIALS EMPHASIZED THAT HUMAN "CONTROLS SHOULD BE CAREFULLY CHOSEN. MINIMUM CONTROLS SHOULD INCLUDE NORMAL INDIVIDUALS OF THE SAME RACE, AGE, AND ENVIRONMENT AS THE PATIENT POPULATION. . . INTERNATIONAL COOPERATION IS HIGHLY RECOMMENDED TO ASSURE THE HOMOGENEITY OF SEROLOGY (i.e. blood testing), DISEASE CLASSIFICATION, AND CHOICE OF APPROPRIATE CONTROL POPULATION."

No clue was given regarding "the population" which would be chosen for human vaccine experimentation. But anyone who knew how secret medical experiments were performed, or who was aware of the third-world activities of the John E. Fogarty International Center for Advanced Study in the Health Sciences, and the World Health Organization, would know who would be selected.

Eleven years later, the John E. Fogarty International Center (along with the NCI, the National Institute of Allergy and Infectious Diseases, and the AIDS Institute of the New York City Department of Health) would provide financial support to bring together the world's best known virologists at a meeting at the Cold Spring Harbor Laboratory. In September 1983, they convened to discuss the "role" of the the human T-cell leukemia/lymphoma virus "family" in the production of human cancer and AIDS. Max Essex dedicated the meeting to Mary Lasker, who "led us to believe in ourselves and to sustain the search for viruses that cause cancer."

A year later, Gallo and Essex presented the green monkey story of AIDS to the scientific world. With their subsequent discoveries of "new" AIDS-like viruses in Africa, the African origin of AIDS was firmly established.

Gallo was confident the AIDS virus arose in Africa "in the bush." But strangely, the bush people were not the ones who were most affected by AIDS. In central Africa, AIDS was a disease of the big cities. The AIDS virus primarily attacked the better-educated class, the blacks who could afford better medical care.

I wondered if Gallo truly believed the theories he was proclaiming; or were his theories promoted to mask effectively a possible "laboratory origin" for the AIDS virus?

The AIDS experts quickly blamed dirty and virus-contaminated needles for the spread of African AIDS. But there was no real evidence for this allegation.

On the contrary, Mads Melbye *et al* tested a large group of patients and workers for AIDS antibodies at a university hospital in Lusaka, Zambia. Their study showed that patients who received many injections were no more likely to have AIDS antibodies than those who didn't. Furthermore, hospital needles were rarely reused. Melbye's team found low rates of antibodies in people over 60 and those under the age of 20. The study concluded that AIDS virus infection "is not widespread throughout the population but is concentrated in the sexually-active age groups, and among persons of higher educational background."

Other AIDS experts claim that scarification rites, and virus-contaminated blood transfusions may be responsible for the high rates of African AIDS, but again there is no proof for these assertions.

AIDS scientists are convinced that the epidemic began in Africa because blood tests have shown that many Africans carry antibodies to the HTLV "family" of viruses. However, some early reports of "positive" AIDS antibody test results in African blood samples were later shown to be in error because of "false-positive" results. It was thought that other frequent African infections, such as malaria and other parasitic diseases, were causing "non-specific" positive test reactions which had nothing at all to do with AIDS virus infection. Some researchers claimed that antibody tests on "old," stored African blood specimens were unreliable because the sera had a "sticky" quality which interfered with the laboratory test results.

In 1986 Karpas and a group of Israeli scientists could not confirm the previously reported "positive" HTLV-1 antibody test results in Africans. Many "positive" HTLV blood test results found by previous investigators were "negative" when retested in Karpas' lab. The Israelis complained that "perhaps the rapid pace of research in this (AIDS virus) area encourages the emergence of spurious claims and the publication of premature data, lacking confirmation and requiring subsequent rebuttal."

Another English and Israeli lab team (Weiss, *et al*) also found inconsistent results in testing African blood. They warned: "Clearly, there is a need to investigate these discrepancies, including exchange of sera between laboratories using different tests."

Despite the "discrepancies" in African blood testing, the theory persists that the AIDS virus had its origins in the steaming jungles of central Africa. And Africans are blamed for starting the epidemic.

Some virologists embellished the monkey theory with lurid details. Norbert Rapoza, a senior virologist employed by the American Medical Association (AMA), was interviewed in the AMA *American World News* (An AIDS expert's grim message, December 5, 1986). Rapoza claims that "AIDS began in central Africa, probably as a monkey virus that jumped species. It may have been spread by mosquitoes that bit rural African tribesmen. Then, the virus may have mutated and when the tribesmen moved to the big cities, two things happened: they became involved with prostitutes and picked up other sexually transmitted diseases, and they were treated for these diseases with dirty needles. So, there were two routes of transmission going on simultaneously — sex and dirty needles. Or the original virus may have come from a hooved animal — a cow or a pig — and may have been transmitted by some African's custom of cutting the neck and drinking the blood."

I was surprised that Rapoza implicated mosquitoes in the African spread of AIDS. The CDC had taken great pains to deny that such a possibility could exist, at least in America.

When gays in New York City showed signs of Kaposi's sarcoma (KS), astute physicians immediately "connected" the so-called "gay cancer" with the serious form of KS which is common in central Africa.

In the central African nation of Uganda, ten percent of all cancer tumors are KS tumors. In children and young African black men, KS can be a highly malignant and rapidly fatal form of cancer. However, in older men KS may persist for many years in a mild form. For an unknown reason, KS is 20 times as common in adult black men than it is in women.

When AIDS broke out in New York City, Los Angeles, and San Francisco, most physicians and scientists naturally assumed that "gay" KS had "something to do" with the highly lethal form of KS common in young African blacks. This assumed "connection" between American and African KS, coupled with the "connection" of the AIDS virus to African green monkeys, became the scientific basis for the belief that AIDS originated in central Africa.

However, after the AIDS virus was discovered, and after the subsequent blood testing of KS cases in Africa, it was discovered that many African KS patients had NEGATIVE AIDS antibody tests!

Although the profound significance of this finding is not generally recognized by most physicians, the implications of these "negative" findings in African KS were perfectly clear to Robert Biggar.

Biggar is an epidemiologist employed by the NIH, who is considered an authority on African AIDS. In the late 1970s, Biggar worked in West Africa, studying Burkitt's lymphoma, (a common cancer tumor in black Africans). In the early 80s, he was involved in U.S. government studies tracing the homosexual spread of the AIDS virus from Manhatten to Denmark, and later tracking the virus from Manhattan to Washington, DC.

His vast epidemiologic experience in America, Europe, and Africa, made him acutely aware of how rapidly the AIDS virus could disseminate from city-to-city and from continent-to-continent.

In an important (but largely overlooked) scientific paper entitled "The AIDS problem in Africa" (*The Lancet*, January 11, 1986), Biggar proclaimed: "THE CLASSICAL, ENDEMIC VARIETY OF KS IN AFRICA IS NOT RELATED TO HTLV-III/LAV (THE AIDS VIRUS) INFECTION."

In plainer terms, Biggar was convinced that the decades-old form of African KS had *no* relationship to AIDS. There was *no* AIDS connection between "gay" KS and African KS because many blacks with KS had *no* antibodies to the AIDS virus.

For the first time, Biggar cast doubt on the purported KS and AIDS "connection" to Africa!

If Biggar was correct, and the AIDS virus was *not*

causing KS in Africa, what was? No one really knew.

Although a decade has passed since the first cases of "gay" KS cancer were discovered, scientists still know nothing about the actual cause of KS. And yet, the myth persists that AIDS experts have brilliantly discovered the "cause" of the epidemic. How could scientists understand AIDS when they knew nothing about KS, the most common form of cancer found in AIDS?

Casting further doubt on the African origin of AIDS, Biggar contended that if AIDS had really existed for a long time in Africa, THE DISEASE WOULD CERTAINLY HAVE BEEN RECOGNIZED!

Biggar's facts did not support the theory that AIDS began in Africa. On the contrary, a careful review of medical records reviewed at Belgian and French-run hospitals in central Africa showed that AIDS BECAME COMMON ONLY AFTER 1980!

Biggar was emphatic in his belief that, "There is no conclusive evidence that the AIDS virus originated in Africa, SINCE THE EPIDEMIC SEEMED TO START AT APPROXIMATELY THE SAME TIME AS IN AMERICA AND EUROPE. The origin of HTLV-3/LAV (the AIDS virus) is of more than historical interest. The AIDS agent, a complicated retrovirus with core proteins and a glycoprotein envelope COULD NOT HAVE ORIGINATED DE NOVO. The identification of the progenitor agent from which this agent either mutated or recombined has significant implications."

Biggar forcefully concluded: "THE ORIGIN OF THE CAUSATIVE (AIDS) AGENT REMAINS UNKNOWN."

As I carefully studied Biggar's paper I began to pick

up little clues that seemed to go along with Strecker's strange ideas about the AIDS happening in Africa. If Biggar was right, and if the AIDS virus didn't originate "de novo" in Africa, where did it come from?

Biggar's use of the Latin term "de novo" meant "anew." The term suggested the AIDS virus did not newly appear out of the blue. Because of its complex and unprecedented molecular structure, the AIDS virus had to have been manufactured, or engineered, or recombined, or born out of some other deadly virus, or "progenitor."

Despite Biggar's puzzling new revelations, the AIDS scientists remained silent on the issues he raised.

AIDS researchers repeatedly insisted the explosion of African AIDS was a result of promiscuity. But in one study, 67% of young black African children showed AIDS virus antibodies. Surely, the scientists weren't blaming promiscuity and anal sex for those test results in children!

Certain AIDS experts claimed the childrens' blood tests might be showing "false-positive" reactions. However, this was not a valid point because the children had the same antibody AIDS test that was used to test African adults. The massive number of AIDS deaths in Africa proved the AIDS antibody test was significant.

I pondered on the WHO "recommendations" to test children ("sibships") with new "antigens" that could be injected along with preventive (childhood) vaccinations. If African children were injected with contaminated human vaccines, as Strecker suggested, this could explain why so many black children were testing positive for AIDS antibodies.

If AIDS had been smouldering in central Africa for years (as so many experts surmised) it would seem logical that old people, rather than children, would have higher high rates of AIDS antibodies. Peculiarly, a Ugandan blood study designed to test this hypothesis showed this was not the case.

In an article entitled "How long has the AIDS virus been in Uganda?" (*The Lancet*, May 24, 1986), J.W. Carswell, *et al* compared AIDS antibody test results in young and old people in Uganda. Carswell's group tested 53 individuals over the age of 70 who were living in geriatric homes in Kampala, Uganda's largest city. All the elderly people were "sexually inactive for the past five years." Their tests were compared to 716 healthy adults also living in Kampala.

Not surprisingly, 15% of the city people were antibody positive. Amazingly, NONE of the elderly people were positive. On the basis of these negative tests, the researchers concluded that the virus had not been in Uganda for a long time. They wrote: "The results presented here do not support previous suggestions that the virus might have originated in Uganda; on the contrary, if interpreted correctly, THEY INDICATE IT ARRIVED IN THE COUNTRY ONLY RECENTLY."

Many Africans deplore the claim of American AIDS experts that AIDS originated in Africa. Instead they insist they are being used as scapegoats for AIDS by racist scientists.

American AIDS experts have also fostered the belief that AIDS entered the U.S. indirectly through Haiti. More specifically, most American scientists believe that promiscuous New York gays brought the AIDS virus back to America from Haiti.

Undoubtedly, there are some sexual AIDS "connections" between Haiti and America. There are white homosexual cases, as well as Haitian-American AIDS cases that can be traced back to "gay" liasons in Haiti. But it is also likely that the theory of a Haitian origin for American AIDS will eventually prove to be another AIDS myth.

Knowledgeable people now understand that the AIDS virus can affect ALL sexually-active persons. Therefore, the purported concept of AIDS being brought to America EXCLUSIVELY by gay men would seem to be not only highly unlikely, but also biologically impossible.

Let us examine why.

THE HAITIAN CONNECTION

The Haitian AIDS connection is still shrouded in mystery because of the inability or unwillingness of U.S. government scientists to initiate AIDS epidemiologic studies in Haiti similar to those conducted in countries like Denmark, and other distant geographic areas of the world.

In 1982, a year after the "official" onset of AIDS, the first reports of AIDS cases in Haitians living in New York City, Newark, and Miami, began to filter into the CDC.

The epidemiology of Haitian AIDS was complicated by the fact that AIDS cases were also discovered in Port-au-Prince, and in the suburb of Carrefour, an area noted for its houses of prostitution.

At the time, American epidemiologists claimed it was

difficult to assess the true extent of Haitian AIDS. There was insinuation of an alleged "cover-up" by the Haitian government, headed by the dictatorial Duvalier family. Despite the eventual ouster of "Baby Doc" Duvalier and his subsequent exile to France, it still appears difficult to determine the extent of AIDS in Haiti. It may be that American scientists do not want to publicize the true facts about AIDS in Haiti because the facts could conflict with the well-established African origin of AIDS.

The discovery of AIDS in Haiti, and in "high-risk" Haitian-Americans, quickly led to a severe crippling of the Haitian tourist trade. U.S. scientists heavily promoted the theory that AIDS was brought to America by affluent, young promiscuous gays from Manhattan, who regularly traveled to Port-au-Prince and Carrefour where it was cheap and easy to have sex with Haitian men. Early in the epidemic, epidemiologists emphasized that AIDS was a homosexual disease acquired by the practice of anal-genital sex. The public was repeatedly informed that the "gay plague" was brought to America by Manhattan gays sodomized in Haiti.

In his AMA interview, Norbert Rapoza (see page 118) further detailed his elaborate theory on the spread of AIDS to America. "One theory of how AIDS migrated from Africa is that some Haitians used to work in Zaire (in central Africa) and had returned by 1977, when an international conference of gays was held in Haiti, where the virus could have been spread by sex or drugs or both and then have been taken back to New York and California." (Despite Rapoza's claim, there is no record of such a "gay" international conference in

Haiti in 1977, or in any other year).

Although AIDS in Haiti is widely believed to have been imported from Africa, Jane Teas of the Harvard School of Public Health presented another theory in 1983. Teas suggested a "connection" between Haitian AIDS and an outbreak of "African Swine Fever Virus" (ASFV) infection which occurred in Haiti in the late 1970s.

According to Teas, ASFV was discovered in Haitian pigs in 1979, a year which correlates with the first AIDS cases in Haiti. She claims the clinical symptoms of swine virus infection (fever, swollen lymph nodes, loss of appetite, and immunosuppression) are similar to the symptoms of AIDS.

The swine fever virus theory of AIDS never attained much credibility in the scientific community, and when the AIDS virus was discovered, the theory was largely abandoned. Nevertheless, a few reporters keep Teas' ASFV theory alive, and have tainted it with insinuations of covert CIA activity in the Caribbean.

In an editorial in the *New York Native,* (February 17, 1986), Charles Ortleb reminded his readers that the CIA had been accused of introducing African swine fever virus into Cuba in 1971. Quoting from a report in the *Boston Globe,* (January 9, 1977), Ortleb wrote: "With the tacit backing of Central Intelligence Agency (CIA) officials, operatives linked to anti-Castro terrorists introduced African swine fever virus into Cuba in 1971. Six weeks later, an outbreak of the disease forced the slaughter of 500,000 pigs to prevent a nationwide epidemic."

After the CIA released the virus in Cuba, Ortleb

surmises the disease spread among pigs in the Caribbean and then spread into South America, paving the way for AIDS virus infection in the late 1970s. *Ortleb believes the AIDS "retrovirus is used by government scientists at the CDC to mask the real (African swine fever virus) cause of AIDS." (The CDC has repeatedly denied that the swine fever virus is involved in AIDS).*

In another *New York Native* story (Haiti: The great AIDS cover-up, April 21, 1986), Anne-Christine D'Adesky again raised the controversial CIA issue by declaring: "If African swine fever virus was linked to AIDS in Haiti, and African swine fever originally broke out in the Caribbean due to a CIA plot, could the U.S. be indirectly implicated for causing and/or spreading AIDS?" D'Adesky surmises that any AIDS theory implicating the CIA would be vigorously suppressed in America.

Although the swine fever virus has not been linked directly to AIDS, it is conceivable that the swine virus could act as a "co-factor" in some AIDS cases. In 1986, Shyh-Ching Lo of the Armed Forces Institute of Pathology in Washington discovered a new and "novel" (and as yet unidentified) virus in the blood of some AIDS cases. This surprising finding raised an important question. Could this "new" virus be the African swine fever virus?

Many Haitians do not believe the American story that blames them for bringing AIDS to the Western Hemisphere. Their strongest argument is the fact that AIDS IN HAITI STARTED ABOUT THE SAME TIME THAT AIDS STARTED IN NEW YORK CITY GAYS. In fact, some Haitians use epidemiologic data to suggest that Manhattan gays brought the disease to Haiti!

The purple skin spots of Kaposi's sarcoma remain the unmistakable "mark" of AIDS. The first case of "fulminant" Kaposi's sarcoma (KS) in a Haitian man was diagnosed in Port-au-Prince in June 1979, the same year the first gay cases were discovered in New York City. This case, along with 61 other Haitians who developed KS and/or opportunistic infections between 1979-1982, was reported by physicians in Haiti in 1983.

The Haitian doctors searched the hospital records but could find only one previous Haitian case of KS who was diagnosed seven years earlier, in 1972. There was no record of any other Haitian case before that year. The new Haitian AIDS cases were young (median age of 32 years), mostly men (85%), and most patients died within six months. One-third of the AIDS cases also had tuberculosis.

Fifteen percent of the men were bisexual. These bisexual men were considered to be an epidemiologic "link" between American and Haitian AIDS cases. According to the Haitian doctors, some men "had had sexual relations with American homosexuals in New York and Miami."

The Haitian physicians emphasized "the first cases of KS and opportunistic infection in Haiti were recognized in 1978-1979, a period that coincides with the earliest reports of AIDS in the United States."

Jeffrey Vieira, *et al* reported on ten of the earliest AIDS cases in Haitian men living in New York City, who were evaluated between January 1981 and July 1982. Vieira's group was surprised to find that none of the Haitians were gay or addicted to drugs. In New York City, what did heterosexual Haitians and homosexual men have in common? Unfortunately, nobody knew. But the CDC quickly declared that Haitians-Americans were at "high risk" for AIDS. The Haitians were a confusing "risk" group who belied the notion that AIDS was a disease of gays and druggers.

New and bizarre theories about Haitian AIDS continue to flourish in the most prestigious medical journals. One persistent story is that Haitians could have been exposed to the AIDS virus during the preparations of "sorcerer's poison" from the brains of dead people, or through the ingestion of "human blood in (voodoo) sacrificial worship." Such notions prompted William Greenfield to write a letter to the Editor, which was published in *JAMA,* (October 24, 1986). The letter was fancifully titled "Night of the Living Dead II: Slow virus encephalopathies and AIDS: Do necromantic zombiists transmit HTLV-3/LAV during voodooistic rituals?"

Almost a decade after the first case of AIDS was discovered in Haiti, the origin of Haitian AIDS remains a mystery. However, no scientist believes the AIDS virus "originated" on the island because AIDS is not a problem in the Dominican Republic, which shares the island of Hispaniola with Haiti.

It is now clear that most AIDS cases in Haiti are heterosexual. Some reports claim that 40% of the cases are women. In this respect, the epidemiology of AIDS in Haiti is more like AIDS in Africa.

If Manhattan gays did bring the AIDS virus into America from Haiti, it is not likely they would have been the EXCLUSIVE recipients of a sexually transmitted virus which spreads so easily between heterosexuals in Haiti.

In 1985 a highly authoratative textbook was published, entitled *AIDS: Etiology, Diagnosis, Treatment, and Prevention*. The book was edited, in part, by Vincent DeVita, Director of the National Cancer Institute.

Two NCI epidemiologists, James Goedert and William Blattner, clarified some details of the Haitian AIDS story. They concluded:

1. There is no evidence that the AIDS virus originated in Haiti, nor is it possible at this time to determine whether homosexual American tourists introduced AIDS into Haiti, or whether they returned from Haiti with the AIDS virus.

2. The incidence of AIDS in Haitians who emigrated to the United States since 1978 is 40 times higher than those who emigrated before 1978.

3. The disease in Haiti is concentrated primarily in Port-au- Prince and Carrefour (the latter area "reportedly being a center of male and female prostitution").

4. As many as one-third of the Haitian men with AIDS may be bisexual or "serve as prostitutes for American tourists."

5. At least one-quarter of Haitian cases are women.

6. There is no evidence that voodoo practices or ingestion of animal blood contribute to the risk of AIDS.

Goedert and Blattner admitted "a complete explanation of the AIDS epidemic may never be possible." They reiterated that the key to AIDS may be the discovery of new AIDS-like viruses in Africa. In 1986, Biggar contradicted this view by presenting his epidemiologic data which cast serious doubt on the African origin of AIDS.

These new details on Haitian AIDS renewed my interest in the underground theory which accuses the CIA of conducting secret biological experiments on male and female Haitian prostitutes in Carrefour. Proponents of this theory insist that prostitutes were deliberately injected with viruses during routine injections of antibiotics for sexually-transmitted diseases. The theory seems so bizarre, and yet there are statistical and epidemiological peculiarites of Haitian AIDS that could be compatible with covert human experimentation.

In this regard, the CIA has a long history of secret drug experiments on unwilling and unsuspecting American civilians. In some of these experiments which have recently come to light, victims were lured to hotel rooms for sexual encounters with prostitutes, and then subsequently drugged and monitored by CIA agents. These government-sponsored experiments which took place in New York, San Francisco, and other cities, are chronicled in *A Higher Form of Killing*. Although most Americans are unaware of these intolerable activities by government agencies, the questionable ethics of the CIA has become known to the public as a result of the Congressional Iran-Contra Hearings in 1987.

Something obviously happened in Haiti around the late 1970s to account for the outbreak of AIDS. Surprisingly, no epidemiologist has ever provided a satisfactory theory to explain why Haitians entering the U.S. after 1978 were FORTY TIMES AS LIKELY TO

GET AIDS. These peculiar statistics of Haitian AIDS are rarely mentioned in the scientific literature. Instead, many AIDS experts, (apparently unaware of the "official" epidemiologic stand on the Haitian issue in DeVita's "AIDS" book), continue to blame gays for bringing AIDS to America.

Undoubtedly, world-traveling heterosexuals must have partaken of the AIDS virus during visits to the famed brothels of Carrefour and Port-au-Prince. Yet it is rare to discover an AIDS case in the scientific literature that was "picked-up" in Haiti and carried to other parts of the world. Unbelievably, only New York City gays were blamed for spreading AIDS.

If AIDS was imported to Haiti from Africa, it is unlikely the epidemic would have broken out in Port-au-Prince and in Manhattan during the same time period (around 1979). If Haitian men were spreaders of the AIDS virus, it would seem reasonable to expect that sexually-active Haitians traveling to New York and Miami would also infect other Haitians living in America. If that were the case, it would seem likely that Haitian-Americans would be the FIRST group to get AIDS in America. But the facts show that cases of AIDS in Haitians living in America were discovered around 1982, three years AFTER the first homosexual cases were discovered in 1979 in New York City.

Another peculiar discrepancy about AIDS is why Haitians were the ONLY nationals in the world who brought AIDS back from Africa. In view of what we now know about the epidemiology and sexual transmission of the AIDS virus, it would seem to be a biologic impossibiity for the Haitians to have accomplished this feat.

Theories on the Haitian — AIDS connection continue to flourish in the media. According to the *Los Angeles Times*, (Male prostitution and the heterosexual community, August 9, 1987), new data suggests that New York City gays brought the AIDS virus to Haiti! This is the new "official" story purported by Jean Pape, a Haitian-born physician "who has been researching AIDS in his hometown of Port-au-Prince since 1982."

In the same article, Ronald St.John of the Pan American Health Organization in Washington also blamed homosexual men for spreading AIDS south of the American border. In his view, "In one country after another, the first case reported was always, always, some local who had traveled to the U.S. and was gay."

Neither Pape nor St. John provided a story to explain how an African AIDS virus could have initially seeded itself exclusively in young gay men living on the island of Manhattan.

No doubt, experts will continue to provide "official" and unofficial theories about Haitian AIDS. It is possible that some day these stories will be among the biggest "fairy tales" ever reported in the medical literature.

On May 11, 1987, *The London Times*, one of the world's most respected newspapers, published an explosive article entitled "Smallpox vaccine triggered AIDS virus." The story suggested that the smallpox eradication vaccine program sponsored by the WHO was responsible for unleashing AIDS in Africa. Almost 100 million black Africans living in central Africa were inoculated by the

WHO. The vaccine was held responsible for awakening a "dormant" AIDS virus infection on that continent.

An advisor to the WHO admitted, "Now I believe the smallpox vaccine theory is the explanation for the explosion of (African) AIDS." Robert Gallo told *The Times*, "The link between the WHO program and the epidemic is an interesting and important hypothesis. I cannot say that it actually happened, but I have been saying for some years that the use of live vaccines such as that used for smallpox can activate a dormant infection such as HIV (the AIDS virus)."

Despite the importance of the story, the U.S. media was silent on the issue. For some strange reason, the story was killed. Reporters like Jon Rappoport spoke to newspeople at the Associated Press in Washington, Boston, and New York; Reuters at the United Nations; and the United Press International in New York. No one he interviewed had ever heard of the story out of London.

It was all very strange — but it went along with what people like Strecker were saying about foul play in Africa. It smelled like another cover-up. The biomedical establishment and the government officials believed in the "green monkey theory" of AIDS — and no damn smallpox vaccine theory was going mess up that established fact.

After meeting and talking with Strecker on many occasions, I began to "read between the lines," and I questioned everything I read in the scientific journals.

AIDS was the medical mystery of the century. The killer had been discovered. It was an ingenious, tiny genetic package of death. A particle that had already infected the bodies of one hundred million people worldwide. The AIDS virus had arisen "de novo," but it had to have originated somewhere. The scientific community laughed at people like Strecker, and others, who said the virus was manufactured.

A new killer AIDS virus had been identified, and no one knew how to stop it. Nobody was laughing about that.

A few people began to wonder how the killer had gotten out. Who was responsible for releasing such a monster? And why would anyone do such a dastardly thing to destroy lovemaking on the planet?

References:

Memoranda. Virus-associated immunopathology: animal models and implications for human disease. 1. Effects of viruses on the immune system, immune-complex diseases, and antibody-mediated immunologic injury. Bull WHO 47: 257-264, 1972.

Memoranda. Virus-associated immunopathology: animal models and implications for human disease. 2. Cell-mediated immunity, autoimmune diseases, genetics, and implications for clinical research. Bull WHO 47: 265-272, 1972.

Fogerty International Center Proceedings N. 15. Biological significance of histocompatibility antigens. Federation Procedings 31: 1087-1104, 1972.

Melbye M, Bayley A, Manuwele JK, et al: Evidence for heterosexual transmission and clinical manifestations of human immunodeficiency virus infection and related condtions in Lusaka, Zambia. Lancet 2:1113-1115, 1986.

Karpas A, Maayan S, Raz R: Lack of antibodies to adult T cell leukemia virus and to AIDS virus in Israeli Falashas. Nature 319:794, 1986.

Weiss RA, Cheingsong-Popov R, Clayden S, et al: Lack of HTLV-I antibodies in Africans. Nature 319:794-795, 1986.

Biggar RJ: The AIDS problem in Africa. Lancet 1, January 11, 1986, pp 79-82.

Carswell JW, Sewankambo N, Lloyd D, et al: How long has the AIDS virus been in Uganda? Lancet 1, may 24, 1986, p1217.

Teas J: Could AIDS agent be a new variant of African swine fever virus? Lancet 1, April 23, 1983, p923.

Lo SC: Isolation and identification of a novel virus from patients with AIDS. Am J Trop Med Hyg 35: 675-676, 1986.

Harris R, Paxman J: *A Higher Form of Killing,* Hill and Wang, New York, 1982.

Pape JW, Liautaud B, Thomas F, et al: Characteristics of the acquired immunodeficiency syndrome (AIDS) in Haiti. New Engl J Med 309: 945-950, 1983.

Vieira J, Frank E, Spira TJ, et al: Acquired immune deficiency in Haitians. Opportunistic infections in previously healthy Haitian immigrants. New Engl J Med 308: 125-129, 1983.

CHAPTER EIGHT

The Pandemic
of AIDS

In 1969, during a Congressional Hearing, it was predicted that a "super germ" could be developed as part of our experimental biowarfare program. Based on new capabilities for biological warfare resulting from recent advances in genetic engineering, such a manufactured super germ could wipe out vast numbers of people — and the infectious agent could be constructed in such as way that human beings would be powerless against it.

A spokesman for the Department of Defense declared that "WITHIN THE NEXT 5 TO 10 YEARS, IT WOULD PROBABLY BE POSSIBLE TO MAKE A NEW INFECTIVE MICRO-ORGANISM WHICH COULD DIFFER IN CERTAIN IMPORTANT RESPECTS FROM ANY KNOWN DISEASE-CAUSING ORGANISMS. MOST IMPORTANT OF THESE IS THAT IT MIGHT BE REFRACTORY TO THE IMMUNOLOGICAL AND THERAPEUTIC PROCESSES UPON WHICH WE DEPEND TO MAINTAIN OUR RELATIVE FREEDOM FROM INFECTIOUS DISEASE. (Testimony before a subcommittee of the House Committee on Appropriations, Department of Defense Appropriations for 1970, Washington, 1969).

137

Several years later in 1973, J. Clemmesen, a Copenhagen epidemiologist, gave a lecture to cancer researchers attending a symposium on leukemia virus research. He spoke of his concern about the transmissibility of cancer-causing viruses, and the future possibility that someday one of these dangerous and infectious viruses could cause a world epidemic of cancer.

Clemmesen visualized "a mutation of a virus into a variety of high contagiosity to man, resulting in a pandemic of neoplastic (cancerous) disease, before we could develop a vaccine." In an obvious reference to germ warfare, the Dane also asked his audience to imagine "the risk of some desperate persons or nations coming into possession of some virus, so that they could threaten to spread their virus unless some requests were fulfilled." He envisioned "top-secret" biological projects and their disastrous consequences.

Cautioning his fellow scientists not to "leave too much of such ideas to science fiction writers," Clemmesen predicted that "we may have to study such problems before too long."

A decade later, Clemmesen's predictions proved accurate when the fantasy of a worldwide epidemic of cancer became the reality of the AIDS epidemic. By the mid-1980s, one hundred-thirteen countries were reporting cases of AIDS, and AIDS became the pandemic that threatened every nation on the planet. WHO statistics indicated that ten million people worldwide were infected with the virus.

A world that could never agree on politics, or religion, or culture, was starting to comprehend that a massive international cooperative effort would be necessary to halt the spread of the new virus.

In January 1987 the Surgeon General, Everett Koop, spoke to a group of 6000 students at Reverend Jerry Falwell's Liberty University in Lynchburg, Virginia. His AIDS predictions were the most ominous ever spoken by a public official.

Koop's manner was straightforward as he calmly told the students that by the end of the century nearly 100 million people throughout the world would die of AIDS. He emphasized the disease "is uniformly fatal. . . and no cure or vaccine is in sight for the forseeable future."

The new reality of AIDS began to cast doubt on the old myths. In truth, the AIDS virus didn't care if you were promiscuous or monogamous. It didn't matter if you were gay or straight, young or old, white or black, smart or dumb, drug-addicted or health conscious. The new dictums were that "good" people with strong religious and philosophical beliefs could die of AIDS. Innocent children were not exempt from the plague.

To get AIDS, the only requirement was to become infected with the new virus. Nothing more; nothing less.

The new statistics supplied by the epidemiologists were beyond belief. The CDC estimated that one in every 30 American men between the ages of 30 and 50 years had antibodies to the AIDS virus. By 1991, five million Americans would be infected with the AIDS virus. There would be a cumulative total of 300,000 cases with 170,000 deaths. By 1996, one million Americans would have full-blown AIDS. And all these statistics were conservative estimates.

These figures for the 1990s did not include people suffering from AIDS-related complex (ARC) or other

AIDS-related diseases. Those illnesses, although potentially fatal, did not fit the CDC's narrow definition of
AIDS, and therefore were not included in the statistics.
Some experts estimated that for every AIDS case there
were 10 cases of AIDS-related complex. And for every
person known to carry the AIDS virus, there were 50
people who carried it but didn't know they had it.

With each passing year of the epidemic, the prognosis
for AIDS virus carriers worsens. Initially, the experts
thought that around 10% might develop full-blown
AIDS. Within a few years, the figure rose to 20-30%.
By 1987, the prevailing scientific belief was that 75% or
more might come down with AIDS.

Future predictions are difficult to make because the
true incubation period of the AIDS virus is still
uncertain. Strecker was convinced that all virus carriers
would eventually die of AIDS or AIDS-related diseases,
and that the incubation period was lifelong.

There are an estimated 1.5 million American "high
risk" intravenous (IV) drug abusers. The prognosis for
this high risk group is gloomy because the AIDS virus
apparently spreads easily from person-to-person during
the drug ritual of needle-sharing. Attempts to discourage
needle-sharing have usually met with failure; and
proposals to hand out free, sterilized needles to addicts
have been thwarted by political, religious, and social
groups.

Savvy addicts have learned a simple and cheap
procedure to dinsinfect their needles and syringes before
use. The injection materials are placed in a small
waterglass. Half the glass is filled with water; the other
half with common household bleach. This easy procedure

effectively kills the AIDS virus.

By the mid-1980s the precise number of AIDS carriers in America was not known. Estimates were that one to two million people had been exposed. In 1985, the military initiated compulsory AIDS-antibody blood testing for all new recruits. The preliminary results of this testing were released by the CDC in August 1986.

Not surprisingly, the youngest recruits had the lowest infection rates. For age 17, positive tests were found in 0.2% per 1000; for age 26, 4.4% per 1000. Men were three times as likely to be positive than women. Recruits from coastal regions of the country (other than New England) and those from large urban centers had the highest rates of infection.

A CDC "update" report, released in December 1986, contained the following data on the first 25,834 AIDS cases. In adults, ninety-three percent of the cases were men. Ninety percent of the men were between 20 and 49 years of age. Sixty-three percent were white; 22%, black; 14% Hispanic. There were 349 children with AIDS. 56% of the adults had died, and 61% of the children. Over 79% of those diagnosed before January 1985 were dead.

In 1987, the CDC provided statistics on AIDS antibody carriers in the high risk groups. Depending on the area of the country, male homosexuals tested 24% to 68% positive, and IV drug abusers 2% to 68% positive. Hemophiliacs were the group most at risk for AIDS with 40% to 88% positive.

At the beginning of the epidemic, scientists and physicians had told the public there was little to fear from AIDS, unless they were "high-risk" gays, Haitians, hemophiliacs, or heroin addicts. But by the late 1980s, the public was slowly made aware that AIDS was no longer a gay disease. Suddenly everyone was "at risk," and twelve million Americans who had had blood transfusions between the years 1978-1985 were asked to get an AIDS antibody test. The panic was just beginning.

Many people, including some physicians, continued to blame gay people for the ever-increasing plague. Steven Hodge, a Houston physician interviewed by *American Medical News*, (November 8, 1985), was adamant in his condemnation of homosexuals. "This perverted group is undermining the family values and moral fiber of this city. They are walking sewers, carrying diseases in their bodies. We need to establish discipline. . . (homosexual) debauchery and perversion threatens the public health. These are evil individuals with anti-social behavior."

More than any other world event in the late twentieth century, the epidemic of AIDS was tearing apart the social, political, and religious beliefs of millions of human beings. There was never a disease that so deeply affected the sex lives of people everywhere.

Never before had there been a sexually transmitted disease that pitted the forces of "good" against "bad," morality against immorality, and heterosexuality against homosexuality. Couples questioned their fidelity as never before; parents turned against their gay children; and even priests shunned their homosexual parishioners.

It was inevitable that the churches and the religions would be brought into the AIDS foray, particularly over the use of condoms to prevent the sexual transmission of the AIDS virus.

The condom issue erupted when AIDS prevention

organizations attempted to bring AIDS prevention education into minority communities. A confrontation developed between the Catholic church and AIDS prevention groups in Los Angeles in late 1986.

The reason for this confrontation had its roots in AIDS statistics which clearly showed that the black and Hispanic communities were suffering disproportionately from AIDS. Although blacks comprise about 10% of the U.S. population, they comprise about one-quarter of the AIDS cases. Hispanics represent 6% of the population, and 14% of the AIDS cases. Together, black and Hispanic men are three times as likely to get AIDS than white men. Black and Hispanic women are 15 times as likely to get AIDS than white women. Higher rates of IV drug use may be partially responsible for these shocking statistics.

AIDS prevention groups have discovered that the dissemination of AIDS prevention information to minorities can be difficult. Part of the reason is that homosexuality and bisexuality are touchy subjects, particularly in Latin cultures. And recommendations of contraceptive devices, such as condoms, are often culturally unacceptable to poor blacks and Latinos.

The issue of condoms in AIDS prevention is a troublesome one, especially for Roman Catholics. Attempts to educate people on the subject of "safe sex" with condoms have angered religious leaders.

Archbishop Roger Maloney recently withdrew church support from AIDS Project Los Angeles when that group attempted to inform the Latino community about condom usage. The Archbishop was widely quoted as saying, "The Roman Catholic church does not approve the use of condoms. In the issue of AIDS, such use implies either heterosexual promiscuity or homosexual activity. The church approves of neither."

The negative reaction of the Catholic Church toward AIDS prevention education surprised many people. However, the Church's hostility towards practicing homosexuals was steeped in centuries of tradition, and was also consistent with current papal policy.

In November 1986, a Vatican "pastoral letter" on homosexuality greatly angered Catholic gays. They were especially incensed that the letter was publically released a few days before the California election to decide on the LaRouche ammendment, calling for the quarantine of persons with AIDS. The Roman Catholic guidelines, approved by the Pope, labeled the practice of homosexuality as an "objective disorder" and "an intrinsic moral evil." In an obvious allusion to the AIDS epidemic, the papal pronouncement condemned homosexuality which could "threaten the lives and well-being of a large number of people." Not only did the pastoral letter anger and sadden Catholic gays, but it also perpetuated the erroneous belief that AIDS was a "gay" disease.

The complex ethical, legal, and moral issues surrounding AIDS blood testing are still unsettled. Some AIDS experts argue that pregnant women should be tested routinely, and that an AIDS blood test should be a mandatory requirement for marriage.

In states like California, AIDS test results must be kept confidential by law. Test results cannot be made public, nor recorded in the medical record. And breach of confidentiality can result in lawsuits.

There is currently great controversy about AIDS testing, and it poses a dilemma for people who have entered new sexual relationships in the 1980s. Without an AIDS test, there is no way of knowing whether a person may be carrying the AIDS virus. For that reason, the use of condoms and/or the avoidance of "body fluid exchange" are advised to prevent transmission of the virus.

There are those who strongly believe that everyone in new sexual relationships should have an AIDS test. However, some people simply cannot handle the psychological trauma of knowing they are positive, or knowing that someone they love is positive. The awful truth is that most people who test "positive" for AIDS antibodies will die in the future from AIDS or AIDS-related diseases. These statistics are very frightening and depressing for most people.

Many marriages of women to hemophiliacs have fallen apart due to the fear of contracting the AIDS virus from their husbands. As mentioned, as many as 88% of hemophiliacs now test positive because they unfortunately received injections of AIDS virus-contaminated plasma used to treat hemophilia.

The extreme fear of AIDS in the gay community is indicated by the results of some sex surveys which now indicate that as many as three out of ten homosexual men practice celibacy. Although celibacy will prevent AIDS in people who have not already been exposed to the AIDS virus, most sexually active people find the practice of celibacy difficult, if not impossible.

Short of celibacy, the sexual transmission of the AIDS virus can be minimized by the practice of "safe sex" and the use of condoms in ALL new sexual encounters.

Safe sex means that body fluids should not be passed between sexual partners during sexual activity. Body fluids include blood, semen, urine, feces, saliva, and women's genital secretions. Oral sex is considered "high-risk" and should be avoided.

The "safest" sex of all is practiced by sexual partners who are both "negative" and who are monogamous. Although this is the scientific and social "ideal," it is hardly the reality, nor is it ever likely to be a reality because of the sexual wanderlust of millions of people.

The answer to the often-asked question of possible AIDS virus transmission in saliva during "deep" kissing is controversial. Deep kissing has been classified as "low risk," and there is no firm evidence that the AIDS virus has ever been acquired solely in this manner.

Studies have shown that passive anal sex without a condom is the most dangerous form of sex, not only for gay men but for anyone engaging in this sexual activity. However, the many AIDS cases in African heterosexuals (who purportedly rarely indulge in anal sex) reemphasize the fact that the AIDS virus can be transmitted through "normal" sexual activity.

In December 1986 a group of doctors reported a case of AIDS in a lesbian who "apparently" acquired the AIDS virus from her drug-using lesbian lover. The virus may have been acquired during oral sex by exposure to vaginal fluids and/or menstrual blood. This lesbian case illustrates the point that all sexually active persons may be at risk for AIDS, even in the absence of a male sexual partner.

Lesbians are currently a "very low risk" group for AIDS, and cases are extremely rare unless the woman has also been a drug abuser. There are still many lesbians who believe they are protected from AIDS because they do not have sex with men. However, lesbians can be infected by bisexual and/or drug-abusing women. In the future, as AIDS virus infection becomes more prevalent in women, we will undoubtedly discover more AIDS cases in lesbians. AIDS transmission in lesbians is also complicated by the fact that many lesbians have had sexual experiences with men.

Homosexual and bisexual women would do well to remember that AIDS in Africa is a heterosexual disease which spreads as easily from women-to-men as from men-to-women. If women can infect men, it is reasonable to assume that women can infect women. The new scientific reality is that AIDS virus carriers can transmit AIDS, regardless of their sexual orientation.

According to the AIDS experts, the only couples who do not have to practice safe sex are those who have been mutually monogamous since 1978, (the probable year the AIDS virus was introduced into America). If one partner has been unfaithful, the rules of safe sex apply.

By the late 1980s, the joys of casual sex that were so heavily espoused in the 60s and 70s had turned into a sexual mine field filled with deadly AIDS virus carriers.

The knowledge gained from AIDS was a triumph for the scientists. As a result, the new gurus of medical science are no longer the physicians. Instead, they are the molecular biologists, the geneticists and the gene splicers, the virologists and immunologists, the biochemists, and a new breed of laboratory biotechnicians.

Their universe is the submicroscopic world of genetic material, and the world of DNA and RNA molecules that compose the building blocks of life itself. A new realm of chromosomes, enzymes, and biochemical reactions that is as incomprehensible to most physicians, as it is to the common man.

It matters little that the new gurus cannot heal people with AIDS. Nor does it seem to matter that they cannot come up with a satisfactory treatment for most forms of cancer. The cure of AIDS and cancer is not their prime concern. They are too busy with other more important priorities and discoveries.

Although the medical profession and the public are confident that this new breed of scientists will soon come up with an effective AIDS vaccine or treatment, the facts reveal otherwise.

The National Academy of Science report, (*Confronting AIDS*, 1986), is clear on the matter. "Developing a vaccine to prevent HIV (AIDS virus) infection and AIDS presents a number of scientific challenges that have never been responded to successfully. As a result, an effective vaccine may be very difficult, if not impossible to produce. A vaccine may not be reasonably expected to be available in less than 5 years. Even for the next 5 to 10 years, the committee generally believes that the probability of a licensed vaccine becoming available is low."

Despite their failure to halt the spread of AIDS, the scientists were progressing and excelling in other areas.

For example, Roger Lewin, writing in *Science*, (July

11, 1986), summed up the results of a Conference on Molecular Biology of Homo Sapiens, which was held at Cold Spring Harbor. Lewin's report reminded me of the virologists and their "mission" at the Biohazards Conference at Asilomar in the early seventies.

According to Lewin, the geneticists are "on the threshold of a new era, one in which humans would become like experimental genetic systems." With the new biotechnology of genetic engineering it is possible "to contemplate mapping and even sequencing, the entire human genome (i.e genetic material)."

I could barely comprehend the rudiments of the new biotechnology, but it was evident that the frightening world of Orwell's *1984* was already here.

The political consequences for humanity can be disastrous if the new genetic technology is used for evil purposes. If diabolic scientists think our genes are not up to par, they can simply snip and splice them to make new ones. Tailor-made, designer genes could be devised that might be more suitable for a government-controlled society — a new kind of master race complete with drones, clones, and slaves. It was the perfect scenario for a Hollywood movie.

Lewin was greatly impressed. "So fast is the development of new understanding and new techniques, that the clinical world is in danger of being left behind." A new Frankenstein monster was being created, and the common man would be powerless to understand it and stop it.

The rise of genetic biotechnology has gone unnoticed by most political groups. A notable exception is the "Green" party in West Germany.

David Dickson, also writing in *Science*, (April 4, 1986), notes that the Greens and other environmental groups fear "the possible application of genetic engineering to humans, which has triggered deep-seated memories of eugenic experiments conducted by the Nazis," as well as concern about the "possible effects of genetically engineered organisms into the environment." Apparently the scientific community has dismissed the Greens' rejection of genetic engineering "as an excessively emotional reaction."

The Greens would undoubtedly turn purple to learn about "Dr. Cloner's Genetic Engineering Home Cloning Kit" ($599), a product designed for teen-agers by an American company called Genemsco. According to *Insight*, (The Washington Times, December 9, 1986), science-minded kids over the age of 12 can easily splice genes and clone common bacteria, like those found in saliva.

Larry Slot, the inventor of the kit, and a former cancer researcher at the Massachusetts Institute of Technology, claims "the equipment and the instructions in the kit allow the child to take a gene from one strain of bacteria that can break down common sugar, and put that gene into another strain of bacteria that normally does not have this capacity." When asked about possible risks, Slot declared, "It is a risk that some kid could create a genetically altered organism that could be potentially dangerous," but such a germ would be "self-limiting since epidemiologists would immediately contain it."

Strecker and I had a good laugh over Dr. Cloner's Kit. We envisioned the newspaper headlines —

"DEADLY VIRUS MADE IN KID'S LAB."

In an interview in the Los Angeles *Daily News*, (November 28, 1986), Dr. David Golde, chief of oncology and hematology at UCLA, and co-discoverer of "HTLV-2" with Robert Gallo, told reporters: "HTLV-1 and HTLV-2 (retroviruses) probably evolved millions of years ago, but to be perfectly frank we don't know where on earth they came from."

In the same article, Dr. Gary Norman of the Norris Cancer Center at USC noted that the AIDS virus seemed to have more in common with certain *animal* retroviruses (lentiviruses) than to Gallo's human retroviruses that caused leukemia and lymphoma cancer. Norman thought the genetic sequences of the AIDS virus and the visna virus were "very much alike."

Norman's concept of the AIDS virus sounded like Strecker's. In Strecker's view, the AIDS virus was made by combining a bovine (cattle) virus with the sheep visna virus. When the two animal viruses combined to make the AIDS virus, it manifested TWO deadly functions: the "bovine" part of the new virus was designed to seek out and destroy T-cells; the "visna" part caused the neurologic and pulmonary symptoms and the wasting of the body that was so characteristic of slow-dying AIDS patients. These were the *same* symptoms that sheep had when they were dying of visna.

I thought about friends and patients who had died of AIDS. The lucky ones died quickly.

For a long time I tried to prove Strecker wrong. Part of me saw his logic, and another part of me was frightened of the madness of his scientific conclusions. Was he an intuitive medical armchair genius — or merely crazy?

At times, I felt like I was playing a part in a fantasy. I was the bumbling Doctor Watson playing to Strecker's ingenious and brilliant Sherlock Holmes. Strecker had carefully put together all the important facts. In the simplest of terms, he presented me with all the scientific clues and deductions that he had garnered from the crime of the century.

After presenting his solution, I imagined him looking at me and declaring, "It's elementary, my dear Watson. Elementary."

Why did I believe in him when so many others thought he was a crackpot? Was there really a conspiracy? Or was it like they all said: a new disease from a monkey virus?

From my vast research over the past three decades, and from reading and studying, I knew there was more to AIDS than a new monkey virus that jumped species. Just as Clemmesen predicted, there was a new pandemic of contagious cancer on the planet. It was a terrifying disease, and it was raging like a forest fire out of control. It would make all previous plagues seem minor in comparison.

The fire was destined to consume millions of people throughout the world. And everyone was so frightened of the conflagration that few people were concerned about who started the fire.

Clemmesen, J: Summation. In, Comparative Leukemia Research 1973, Leukemogenesis, Bibl Haematol, No. 40, Ito Y, and Dutcher RM (Eds), Univ Tokyo Press, Tokyo/Karger, Basel, pp 790-792, 1975.

CDC: Human T-lymphotropic virus type lll/ Lymphadenopathy-associated virus antibody prevalence in US military recruit applicants. JAMA 256:975-977, 1986.

CDC: Update. Acquired immunodeficiency syndrome — United States. JAMA 257:433-441, 1987.

Marmor M, Weiss LR, Lyden M, et al: Possible female-to-female transmission of human immunodeficiency virus. Ann Int Med 105:969, 1986.

Lewin R: Molecular biology of Homo sapiens. Science 233:157-158, 1986.

Dickson D: Gene-splicing debate heats up in Germany. Science 232:13-14, 1986.

CHAPTER NINE

The Politics of AIDS

Many people think medical science is "pure." But in reality, the study of medicine is saturated with politics, and what passes for "medical science" is often a reflection of medical politics. This is particularly true for AIDS.

Unfortunately, the science surrounding the new epidemic is so polluted by social, cultural, economic, and religious judgments, that AIDS has become a metaphor for an unloving and uncaring society.

The future containment of the epidemic will largely depend on our willingness to provide high quality AIDS prevention information to every person in our society. In addition, we must be willing to give persons with AIDS and AIDS-related diseases the care and emotional support they so desperately need.

In this process, we must set aside the political inertia that has allowed AIDS to become the most serious biological holocaust of our time.

The stigmatization of persons with AIDS in America is overwhelming. In general, our society judges people with AIDS as promiscuous, immoral, perverted, and drug-oriented. As a result, AIDS patients are often shunned like lepers in previous centuries.

155

Until now, male homosexuals in large urban centers have borne the brunt of the epidemic, and gays will continue to be the group most severely affected by AIDS for the next decade. It is estimated that half the gay men in large American cities will be dead of AIDS in the 1990s.

For gays, the issue in AIDS is genocide, pure and simple.

At the present time, prostitutes, drug abusers, Haitians, hemophiliacs, Blacks, and Latinos are the groups at highest risk. Half of the children with AIDS are black; 25% are Hispanic.

Most people who are now dying of AIDS are members of the most detested minority groups in America. How Americans will provide care for these unfortunates will determine our worth as a caring society. With the epidemic we face a political and social agenda of enormous magnitude.

Not everyone in our society is displeased with the mass deaths from AIDS. Already the epidemic has been welcomed by racists, homophobes, and those "religious persons" who believe that the punishment for sin is death.

The recorded history of the decade-old epidemic attests to the inability of the medical and scientific establishment to halt the spread of the disease. In the early 1980s, few people outside the gay community recognized the seriousness and magnitude of the AIDS problem. Consequently, the new disease evoked little interest in the medical community. AIDS was initially believed to be a disease of gays and drug addicts, and the experts told the public that "normal" heterosexuals had little to fear. As a result, little was done in terms of AIDS research, prevention, and education.

Over two and one-half years elapsed between the time the first AIDS cases appeared in New York City and the time these cases were reported "officially" in the summer of 1981. In the beginning the disease was widely assumed to have something to do with semen, sodomy, drugs, and a promiscuous "gay lifestyle."

The original and unbelievable scientific ignorance about the true seriousness of the disease has led to the fact that there are now an estimated 500,000 New Yorkers already infected with the AIDS virus. It is predicted that as many as one-half of these people will die from AIDS by the end of this century.

When gay men in New York City, Los Angeles, and San Francisco, began to die by the hundreds, their pleas for help and assistance with this horrible disease went unheeded by the government for over three years. No money was given for AIDS research or AIDS prevention because the disease was not considered to be a major health problem. By 1984 in New York City, AIDS was the leading cause of death for men aged 30 to 39 years; and the second leading cause of death for women aged 30 to 34 years.

By the time the politicians and scientists seriously decided to declare war on AIDS in 1985, the damage had already been done.

A decade after AIDS, larger social, economic, and political issues have now come to the fore. Unfortunately, many of these issues are still being ingnored by politicians, just as they were ignored at the beginning of the epidemic.

For example, who is going to pay for the medical care of AIDS patients? Many health insurance plans are refusing to pay these expenses.

Where will we house the thousands more who will die soon of this catastrophic illness?

Many gays and other high risk people are not covered by insurance, or are no longer able to get insurance due to their "lifestyle." Insurance companies, whose prime concern is making a profit, don't want to insure gays. The medical costs for an AIDS patients now average about $150,000 or more. The only FDA-approved AIDS drug costs up to $13,000 per year per patient. Insurance companies are not anxious to pay these bills for high risk people.

In America we do not have an adequate health care system to meet the medical needs of ordinary illnesses, let alone the hundreds of thousands of future AIDS cases who will die before the end of this century. It is estimated that 40 million Americans have no health insurance, and many hospitals routinely refuse to care for indigent people.

The issue of AIDS blood testing must also be settled. Many people claim that mandatory testing, followed by quarantine of "positive" people will stem the tide of AIDS. However, AIDS testing is a highly volatile political, social, moral, medical, economic, and ethical issue. *And the AIDS blood tests are not always accurate.*

Whom do we test? High risk people, or everyone? Will the test be compulsory? Who will pay for the testing?

It is imperative that we protect the civil rights of

those who test positive, *before* any of these issues can be resolved. At present, gays and other minorities comprise the groups most likely to test positive. It is absolutely necessary that these people be fully protected from the discrimination which could easily result from a government policy of mandatory AIDS-antibody testing.

In a *Los Angeles Times* Poll (July 31, 1987), 42% of Americans would limit "civil rights" in order to control the AIDS epidemic. 19% were "unsure." About half of those polled favored mandatory testing for high-risk groups. Three out of ten persons were in favor of tattooing AIDS virus carriers.

Unlike most Americans, gays lack civil rights. At present, it is illegal to be a practicing homosexual in 24 states and in the nation's capital. Depending on the law, a gay person can be fined as little as $200 (and recorded as a sex offender), or be imprisoned for up to 20 years for homosexual activity. As a result of these archaic laws and punishments, it is impossible to protect the civil rights of gay people under existing statutes.

There are those who insist that quarantine is necessary for AIDS patients and for people who test positive. Some persons advocate the establishment of "concentration camps" for this purpose. But how could society quarantine and provide for 2 million, or 10 million projected future cases? Even if this were possible, the cost would be incalculable.

We live in an American society that largely ignores an increasing number of homeless and mentally disturbed people who roam the streets of every large American city. If we care little for these people, how could we possibly quarantine and restrict the activities of millions of healthy and sick people suspected of carrying the AIDS virus?

Unlike those who carry TB and syphilis germs, persons testing positive for AIDS antibodies are presumed to be infectious for life. Originally, experts thought that people carrying the AIDS virus would develop the disease within two or three years at the most. But in closely following the fate of large groups of gay men who test positive, scientists have now discovered that more cases of AIDS develop five years AFTER exposure to the virus than before five years. This indicates the incubation period for AIDS is very long. It is possible it could take 20 years or more for "healthy" people to become ill after testing positive for AIDS-antibodies.

AIDS quarantine is unworkable and unnecessary because there is no treatment or cure. The disease is not spread by casual contact, and the incubation period is lifelong.

What are we doing to educate ALL Americans NOW to avoid AIDS? At present, many people continue to regard AIDS as a gay disease because the experts initially told them it was a gay disease. As a result, most heterosexuals still think they are safe from the AIDS virus. Through political and scientific double-talk, we perpetuate the myths of "high risk" groups for AIDS. We have failed to convince the public that most sexually-active adults are at risk for AIDS virus infection.

Moralists claim that celibacy and monogamy will prevent AIDS. Monogamy will certainly prevent AIDS if practiced with a sexual partner who is antibody-negative. But monogamy could be fatal if practiced with someone carrying the AIDS virus.

How many sexually-active Americans have been monogamous since 1978 (the year chosen by the CDC as the start of AIDS)? And how many monogamous individuals have a sexual partner who has also been monogamous since 1978?

No one knows the true statistics in America, but I would estimate that "mutual monogamy" would not be a proper label for most long-term sexual relationships, married or otherwise. With the present AIDS crisis, it might be helpful to stop talking about "monogamy and promiscuity," and to start talking about the real sex life of modern Americans.

In America, millions of teenagers engage in sex. Each year, almost one and one-half million teens become pregnant. Four out of five are unmarried; half a million seek abortions.

Every four seconds, an American becomes infected with venereal disease. The unbelievable sexual spread of the AIDS virus in so short a time to an estimated half-million New Yorkers is an indication that mutual monogamy is not widely practiced.

Many leading politicians currently believe that the best way to halt the spread of the epidemic is to "just say no." They urge parents to play a major role in AIDS education by teaching their children the virtues of virginity and celibacy before marriage.

A poll on Teen-Age Sex in *People* magazine (April 13, 1987) seems to have shattered additional political and social myths by revealing the following data.

According to *People*, the average teenager begins to have sex at age 16. By high school graduation, fifty-seven percent of the students have lost their virginity. Over 60% of sexually-active teen-agers do not use contraceptives, and over half of the parents of teens rarely or never talk to them about sex. A mere 15% of college students say that AIDS has caused them to change their sexual behavior. As proof that AIDS education is still in the Neanderthal period, most college students still believe that AIDS is primarily a gay disease.

The truth about American sexuality is that most people are saying "yes" to sex, and that most sexually-active people are ignoring the AIDS epidemic.

In the near future, as AIDS infection becomes more prevalent in heterosexuals, it is likely that medical authorities will demand blood testing for AIDS antibodies. A 1985 *JAMA* editorial (The age of AIDS: A great time for defensive living) by George Lundberg, may be predictive of future trends. Lundberg warns that, "People who are infectious must stop copulating indiscriminantly." However, he readily admitted, "The chances of this change occurring, given our free society and sexual drives, seems almost nil."

Lundberg recommends that women who are carrying the AIDS virus should not get pregnant, and that "we should not engage in sexual activity (oral, anal, or vaginal) with someone who has the AIDS virus." He also considers the value of AIDS virus testing as a requirement for a marriage license, and concludes that "this is a great time to practice sexual monogamy."

In June 1987, the AMA issued its recommendations for MANDATORY AIDS testing of all U.S military personnel, foreign immigrants, blood and tissue donors, and all inmates of federal and state prisons. *Routine* voluntary testing was suggested for patients at VD clinics and drug-abuse clinics, and for pregnant women. In addition, all surgical patients should be tested. If declined, "the hospital and medical staff should consider implementing a *mandatory* program." Voluntary testing was recommended for all IV drugs users, homosexuals and bisexuals, and sexual partners of anyone in these groups.

The fate of prisoners who tested positive was dismal. Naturally, this group was composed primarily of IV drug users and gays. In the future, all federal inmates infected with the AIDS virus would be transferred to the U.S. Medical Center for Federal Prisons in Springfield, Missouri. Despite rampant homosexuality and forced rape in the prisons, the prison officials decided to withhold condoms from all inmates in order not to condone sex acts between men. By this "moral" decision, officials were insuring the spread of the AIDS virus in their institutions. It was a covert and effective way of "cleaning out" the jails with the genocide of prisoners. It was another indication of how murder can be justified by Christian ethics.

By mid-1987, there were more than 22,000 AIDS deaths in the United States. The increasing numbers of American AIDS cases has alarmed other nations, especially those with American military bases.

In February 1987, the Philippine government was shocked when 44 prostitutes tested positive for AIDS-antibodies. Thirty-seven had worked exclusively around

Clark Air Force Base, and Subic Bay Naval Base. In West Germany, a former American army sargeant was arrested in Nuremburg on charges of spreading AIDS to his sexual partners.

Because of the increasing number of cases in Kenya, especially in prostitutes, the British decided to place Kenyan oceanside resorts "off-limits" to military personnel. In India, government-ordered AIDS testing of African students caused an outcry of racism.

Korea, fearing an influx of AIDS with the Seoul 1988 Olympics, has required AIDS testing before issuing resident visas to foreigners. Japan and China are also making plans to keep out foreigners with AIDS antibodies.

Other nations clearly do not want their populations exposed to the American and African epidemic. Undoubtedly, more stringent international health codes and regulations will be imposed in the near future to prevent this from happening.

By the late 1980s, there was little doubt that the AIDS epidemic was becoming synonymous with genocide, at least for gays and black Africans. Historically, mass murder was nothing new. Mankind has always found it easy to justify murder of large groups of people who were hated for various religious, cultural, and political reasons.

In my lifetime, Hitler tried to exterminate all the European Jews, and almost succeeded. In the early 1900s, the Turks systematically killed off 4.5 million Armenians. In Russia, Stalin allowed millions of peasants to starve to death during the years of his unrelentless political purges. In World War II, a hailstorm of atomic bombs in 1945 would have annihilated the Japanese population had they not quickly surrendered. In the 1970s the political regime in Cambodia executed millions of its citizens, including most of its educated class. During the Chinese revolution under the leadership of Mao Tse Tung, fifty million "reactionaries" were eliminated.

In our own bloody history we had only to remember the extermination of the American Indian, the enforced slavery of African blacks, and the internment of 112,000 west coast Japanese-Americans during World War II.

If AIDS is eventually proven to be mass murder through biological warfare, it certainly wouldn't be a new experience for the planet.

The history of biological warfare goes back to World War I when over 180,000 soldiers were gassed by the Germans on the battlefields of Europe. Since that time, biowarfare has been perfected to the point where even greater masses of people can be killed without firing a shot or destroying a building.

Shortly after the war in 1919, Fritz Haber, the German "father" of chemical warfare, received a Nobel Prize for his scientific achievements in chemistry. Since that time, the science of "offensive" biowarfare has been perfected to the point where millions of people can be selectively killed by genetically engineered infectious disease agents designed only for death.

In the 60s and 70s, tens of thousands of young American men were sent to die in Vietnam in a war whose purpose we still do not comprehend. During the war, as part of the government chemical warfare program, the military sprayed the Vietnam earth with a toxic defoliant herbicide known as "agent orange." Many of our young soldiers were exposed to this cancer-causing agent. Later, on returning home, some Vietnam vets developed peculiar and fatal forms of cancer. Some of their children were born with strange birth defects. In the minds of many vets there was little doubt that toxic exposure to agent orange was at the root of their tragic illnesses and family misfortunes.

Predictably, the government denied any wrongdoing. Government doctors and scientists could not uncover "proof" that agent orange was toxic to human beings. In 1984 the vets filed a $1.8 billion class action lawsuit against the federal government. As expected, the trial was characterized by all sorts of legal manuevers, and the case was forcibly settled for $180 million in 1985. So far, the 245,000 vets who are plaintiffs in the case have not received a penny due to pending legal appeals.

Undoubtedly, there are many Americans who would deny that our government would deliberately subject people to dangerous substances, and use them as experimental animals. But in fact, in a story exposing the abuses of biological warfare, the *Los Angeles Times*, (December 4, 1984) cited over 239 U.S Army biowarfare experiments in which unsuspecting civilians and military personnel were used as subjects. Occasionally, details of one of these horror stories comes to light.

For example, in a lawsuit settled in May 1987, U.S. District Judge Constance Baker Motley awarded $700,000 to the estate of Harold Blauer, a 42 year-old mental patient who died in 1953 as a direct result of a series of injections in an Army secret drug experiment performed at the New York State Psychiatric Institute.

In December 1952, Blauer was hospitalized at the mental institution for depression. Although he knew he was receiving an experimental drug, he had no idea he was being used as an unwilling victim in an Army experiment to develop chemical warfare agents.

According to the *Los Angeles Times*, (May 6, 1987), hallucinogenic drugs "were administered to Blauer as part of a classified contract the state-run institute had with the Army Chemical Corps for evaluating the effects of potential chemical warfare agents." He died "as a guinea pig in an experiment to test potential chemical warfare agents for the U.S. army."

In the trial there was evidence of tampering with the medical records, making it "appear that Blauer's death, while triggered by the injection, was really caused by a weak heart."

In a sharply-worded opinion, Judge Motley detailed a "20-year conspiracy" by the Army, the Justice Department, and the New York state attorney general's office to conceal events surrounding the death of Harold Blauer.

I could only wonder how many other Americans have died and will continue to die as a result of secret, government-approved experiments.

Twentieth century human experimentation by physicians is not limited to Jewish victims incarcerated in Nazi concentration camps. In America, one of the most notorious medical experiments involved a group of poor, illiterate black men with syphilis in Macon County, Alabama, who were enrolled in a federal government study during the years 1932-1972.

In the experiment, about 400 black syphilitic share-croppers were examined yearly by Public Health Service doctors in Tuskegee. The purpose of the study was to record the destructive effects of untreated syphilis, and to follow closely the medical progress of the group until each man died.

The black men were never told they had syphilis, nor were they told their disease could endanger their families. They only knew they were being examined yearly and were receiving free treatment for "bad blood," (a term used in the black community to denote a variety of different illnesses).

Even when a penicillin treatment cure for syphilis became available in the 1940s, the men in the Tuskegee Syphilis Experiment were not allowed to receive the antibiotic. By decree, other doctors in Macon County were forbidden to treat any of the men in the study. Only special government doctors could treat the men, and when any of them died, the government quickly made arrangements for autopsy examination at Andrew Hospital.

Autopsies were imperative to assess the pathologic damage caused by the deadly syphilis germs which were allowed to proliferate in the black mens' bodies. As a financial incentive for the men and their families, the government picked up the tab for "burial expenses."

The original scientists who devised and conducted the experiment were convinced that the effects of syphilis in blacks were different than in whites. The Tuskegee experiment was undertaken to prove that hypothesis. Over the years, many medical studies involving these untreated syphilitic men were reported in scientific journals.

During the Black civil rights movement of the 60s, pressure was put to bear on the CDC to stop this inhumane experiment. But despite criticism from a few outspoken people, the government study continued until it was finally disbanded under political pressure in 1972.

An article by Martin P. Levine (Bad blood, *New York Native*, February 16, 1987) examined the racist science inherent in the study. He reminded his readers that the Tuskegee experiment was supervised by the CDC, the same government agency that now oversees the AIDS epidemic.

According to Levine, the experiment was easily justified by physicians and scientists because "it was widely believed that black racial inferiority made them a 'notoriously syphilis-soaked race.' Their smaller brains lacked mechanisms for controlling sexual desire, causing them to be highly promiscuous. They matured early and consequently were more sexually active; and the black man's enormous penis with its long foreskin was prone to venereal infections. These physiological differences meant the disease must affect the races differently."

Levine concluded by reminding his readers that "what happened in Macon County means we cannot blindly trust the CDC. While none of us feels that AIDS is a repeat of Tuskegee, it is high time we took a long hard look at what they are doing. The message from Macon County is simply: Be wary, be critical."

Unbelievably, the diabolic Tuskegee experiment was sanctioned by the American scientific community for five decades. Even the black doctors at Andrew Hospital kept quiet about what was going on right under their noses. Nobody wanted to cause trouble. In this democracy, it is common knowledge that the "whistle blowers" often suffer more than the people they expose.

The experiment could not have been successful were it not for Nurse Eunice Rivers, a black Public Health nurse who watched over the men, and who became their confidante for the duration of the study. She, more than anyone, got the men and their families to cooperate fully with the government doctors. In 1958, Nurse Rivers received the highest commendation awarded by the Department of Health, Education, and Welfare: The Oveta Culp Hobby Award, handed out to the department's most distinguished employee.

Nurse Rivers never felt any qualms about her role in the experiment. In *Bad Blood*, (the definitive account of the Tuskegee study), James H. Jones writes: "She saw herself as a good nurse, one who always did what the doctors ordered." She never considered she was morally wrong by not suggesting that the men receive penicillin for their syphilis. "As a nurse, I didn't feel that was my responsibility. As a nurse. . . we were taught that we never diagnosed; we never prescribed; we followed the doctor's instructions."

When the government finally ended the experiment after 40 years, it was discovered that fifty surviving wives and twenty surviving children were infected with syphilis. They received treatment and compensation for the damage they sustained.

There was never any formal apology recorded anywhere in the medical and scientific literature for this shameful racist experiment. Apologies are rarely appropriate for inclusion in such literature. After all, how do you scientifically measure "feeling," and how do you get "controls," and how do you ask for forgiveness. A peer-review committee is not expected to allow that sort of drivel into their respected journals. That was sentiment, not science.

In March 1987, the American AIDS team headed by Gallo, and the French team headed by Montagnier, finally resolved their legal dispute regarding the "discovery" of the AIDS virus and the patent rights to the AIDS antibody test. President Ronald Reagan finally broke his seven-year silence on the AIDS epidemic by announcing the settlement.

It was agreed that the American and French team would share the patent on the AIDS test, and that each would contribute 80 percent of the royalties to establish an international AIDS research foundation. Strecker and I assumed that Gallo and Montagnier would head the foundation. That way both research teams would stand to lose nothing.

The reason for the settlement was not readily apparent, but scientific sources intimated that the results and reports on the original AIDS virus research were doctored. Hints of scandalous misdoings were suggested by the assertion that "copies" of some scientific documents differed in content from the "original" documents. Already, Gallo had received highly critical disapproval when it was discovered he mistakenly used photographs of Montagnier's AIDS virus in a published paper which presented the photos as Gallo's own virus.

Undoubtedly, a continuation of the lawsuit might bring to light all sorts of improprieties of AIDS research, and might damage the reputation of certain AIDS scientists.

Details of the Franco-American legal controversy appeared in an article by Steve Connor (*New Scientist*, February 12, 1987). The report emphasized that the American and the French virus were "practically identical," leading Connor to speculate that Gallo's AIDS virus might actually be Montagnier's French virus! Connor's story also raised questions about Gallo's scientific credibility. Could the French AIDS virus that Montagnier sent to Gallo on two occasions in 1983 have somehow contaminated Gallo's own isolates? Could Gallo have grown Montagnier's virus in his T-cells? If so, did Gallo get credit for a discovery that was not his? If the "contamination" with the French AIDS virus was deliberate, did someone cheat in Gallo's laboratory?

New Scientist also mentioned errors in Gallo's "discovery" of a new "human" HL23 virus in 1975, that subsequently turned out to be *three different contaminating ape viruses* (gibbon-ape virus, simian sarcoma virus, and baboon endogenous virus). Gallo still cannot account for the contamination, claiming that the whole thing was "bizarre."

Personally, I was becoming increasingly skeptical of AIDS science, and weary of AIDS politics. It was apparent that unless you were one of the big boys or girls on a government research team, you wouldn't be let into the game.

There was a government party line that seemingly made AIDS science very simple. There was a "new" virus that was the "sole" cause of AIDS, and there was an antibody test for this virus. The cure for AIDS would come from a preventive vaccine, or from a drug that would kill or inhibit the virus. That was all there was to it.

The government scientists were entrusted to fix AIDS, and any opposition to their ideas would be suppressed. Nothing would be tolerated that would cast doubt on the medical brilliance surrounding the science of AIDS. The public was nervous about AIDS, and there was no point in upsetting them more than they already were.

It has always been easy to suppress alternative ideas in medical science that are contrary to current scientific dogma. While it is true that most important discoveries can find publication in one of the many scientific journals, it is also a fact that few people in science are likely to read about it unless the discovery is published in one of the top-rated journals. Ironically, the original discovery and report of Montagnier's French AIDS virus were largely ignored, while Gallo's supposedly "different" AIDS virus was enthusiastically received by the AIDS experts.

Controversial ideas in medicine are often disregarded if they do not go along with the status quo. Furthermore, controversial studies and discoveries are rarely "cited." As a result, they quickly become "buried in the literature," unlikely to be resurrected except by open-minded researchers.

Sadly, the average doctor spends about ninety minutes a week reading medical material. The reading often consists of perusing commercially-inspired or drug company-oriented throwaway magazines and newspapers that flood the desks of medical practitioners. If an article does not appear in a specialty journal, or in one of the top journals such as *New England Journal of Medicine, JAMA, Lancet,* or *Science,* it will be read by very few professionals, and will rarely be cited by the media.

Medical and scientific journals are highly political. An editor will rarely allow publication of an article which conflicts with the interests of its editorial board, or with established medical dogma, or with the paid advertisements of the pharmaceutical companies.

For example, a scientific journal formerly called *AIDS Research* is now called *AIDS Research and Human Retroviruses.* The editorial board consists of several dozen cancer and AIDS experts, who are primarily genetic engineers or scientists from government-funded medical institutions. Gallo, Essex, and Montagnier are all on the Board, along with one Board member from a pharmaceutical company. Not surprisingly, the drug company is Burroughs-Wellcome which manufactures AZT, the $13,000 per year drug which is the only FDA-approved medication for AIDS. IT IS UNLIKELY THAT A SCIENTIFIC PAPER ANTAGONISTIC TO ESTABLISHED AIDS RESEARCH COULD EVER FIND ITS WAY INTO THIS JOURNAL.

Currently, AIDS research that does not conform to the idea of the AIDS virus as the "sole" cause of AIDS is not likely to be published anywhere. In addition, anything that smacks of "holistic" and "alternative" treatment for AIDS would rarely, if ever, be published in a top medical journal.

In general, any AIDS organization or AIDS research study that is government-funded must conform to the party line. Even though there is great opposition in the gay community to certain government AIDS policies, it is rare to find a government-funded gay group or organization that will speak out against government science or government scientists.

The same holds true for minority AIDS prevention groups. Many alternative groups who have received government funding have been disheartened to find that the government subsequently becomes the ultimate authority in determining the hiring, the firing, and the policy making decisions of the group.

The irony of the idea that the cure for AIDS lies in a vaccine, or a new drug, should be apparent to those who have studied the history and politics of cancer. Human cancer has been epidemic for a century. Yet we have no effective drug, no vaccine, no cure, and no cause for most forms of cancer.

How can we expect these same scientists who have failed miserably in the treatment of cancer to come up miraculously with a magic bullet for AIDS? And unless something originates with these official bureaucratic scientists, they will ignore it.

If veterinarians cannot prevent, treat, or cure animal cancer with vaccines, how can we expect a cure for AIDS, or cancer, with a vaccine? The sad fact is that veterinarians who have been infecting animals with AIDS and cancer viruses are unable to heal the diseases they create.

There is now little doubt that the bovine leukemia virus of cattle is closely related, if not identical, to the AIDS-like "HTLV-1" virus.

What do veterinarians do with cattle that are infected with this virus? According to a popular textbook on molecular biology (*RNA Tumor Viruses,* 1984, page 942), "eradication programs have relied on detection of high-incidence herds and implementation of slaughter policies." Hopefully, our AIDS scientists will never propose such a recommendation for human beings with AIDS.

Interestingly, there is no vaccine for the prevention of cattle viruses, nor is there yet a vaccine for the common virus-caused skin wart. If scientists can't produce a vaccine for the wart virus, how can they possibly produce one for the AIDS virus?

By 1988, scientists were still blaming "green monkeys" for the most dangerous biological holocaust ever unleashed on this planet. Very few people understood that we had unleashed it ourselves.

It was also apparent the scientists weren't going to come up with an AIDS cure. They were clever at making diseases, not curing them.

The scientists kept insisting they needed an "animal model" in order to better study AIDS. They constantly complained of lack of funds for AIDS research.

Strecker insisted the veterinarians already had an animal model for AIDS when they experimentally produced an AIDS-like disease in two baby chimpanzees in the early 1970s.

In a paper published in *Cancer Research* in 1974, scientists proved you could make viruses "jump" species and produce "new" diseases that had never been seen before. All you needed was government research money.

In the experiment, a team of veterinarians working under a grant from the U.S. Department of Agriculture, took six newborn chimpanzees away from their mothers as soon as they were born. Instead of mothers' milk, the chimps were weaned on milk from another species — the milk of cows who were infected with "bovine C-type virus."

Seven months later, one baby chimp became ill. A month after that, another chimp became sick. Both were lethargic and wouldn't eat. Laboratory tests showed they were suffering from anemia, and their white blood cell counts were elevated. Within six weeks both chimps developed pneumonia and died. The other four animals stayed healthy.

At the autopsy of the two chimps that died, the pathologists found cancerous cells in the bone marrow, spleen, and lymph nodes. All the vital organs of the immune system were damaged, and cancer cells were also found in the liver, lungs, and kidneys.

The doctors were pleased. The two chimps had received the milk of a special cow that was a "reliable and abundant source of bovine C-type virus."

The experiment was a great success. The vets were astounded that they had produced not one, but *two* new diseases in chimpanzees.

The first disease was leukemia — a cancerous disease of the blood stream. The second disease was a parasitic, opportunistic lung infection called *Pneumocystis carinii* pneumonia. PNEUMOCYSTIS PNEUMONIA AND LEUKEMIA HAD NEVER BEEN SEEN IN CHIMPS BEFORE!

A few years later, *Pneumocystis carinii* pneumonia and an infection with a mysterious virus would begin to take the lives of immunodepressed, young gay men in

Los Angeles. Doctors had never diagnosed this infection in previously healthy men; only in debilitated cancer patients had physicians observed death from *Pneumocystis carinii* pneumonia.

The "new" disease in humans was called AIDS. Pneumocystis pneumonia was its hallmark, along with cancer in the form of Kaposi's sarcoma.

The veterinarians were strangely silent on AIDS. This was understandable. AIDS was a human disease, not an animal disease. Only Max Essex of Harvard suspected that one of his "leukemia-lymphoma" animal viruses might be the culprit. His pussy cat experiments in the 1970s proved how deadly AIDS-like viruses could be. And Essex and Donald Frances (who conducted the hepatitis B vaccine trails on the west coast in gay men in 1980) had predicted in 1979 that similar viruses would someday be implicated in the cause of human cancer.

When Essex co-discovered the AIDS virus with Gallo, both men theorized the AIDS virus "family" originated in central Africa, perhaps millions of years ago. Gallo wrote that sixteenth-century Portugeese traders could have picked up the virus in the steaming jungles of Central Africa and brought it to southern Japan where it lay dormant for four centuries until the late 1970s.

Gallo apparently derived his "intriguing" theory from James Clavell's best-selling 1975 novel, *Shogun,* which was referenced in Gallo's October 22, 1983 letter to *The Lancet*. As I recalled from the *Shogun* TV miniseries, the Japanese did not take too kindly to the Portugeese. I could hardly imagine them sleeping with their women. Strecker and I wondered why the Portugeese didn't bring the monkey virus to their other outposts in Asia, and why they didn't bring it back to their wives and lovers in Portugal.

Gallo also thinks, "It seems likely that the origin of HTLV-1 in the Caribbean, the U.S., and South America was from entry of infected Africans to the Americas." A year later, he claimed HTLV-3 was brought in from Africa by the Haitians, and that the virus was brought back from Haiti by traveling New York City gays.

AIDS science was all very simple.

The virus "jumped species" from monkey to man. Within seven years, it was decimating the gay communities in large American cities, and decimating blacks in central Africa.

Strecker believed the AIDS virus came from a lab.

But no AIDS expert would ever admit to story like that.

A story like that would never be found in an American scientific journal.

The whole idea was insane.

References:

Lundberg GD: The age of AIDS: A great time for defensive living. JAMA 253:3440-3441, 1985.

Jones JH: *Bad Blood: The Tuskegee Syphilis Experiment*, The Free Press, New York, 1981.

McClure HM, Keeling ME, Custer RP, et al: Erythro-leukemia in two infant chimpanzees fed milk from cows naturally infected with the bovine C-type virus. Cancer Research 34:2745-2757, 1974.

Gallo RC, Sliski A, Wong-Staal F: Origin of human T-cell leukaemia-lymphoma virus. Lancet 2:962-963, 1983.

Connor S: AIDS science stands on trial, New Scientist, February 12, 1987, pp 49-58.

CHAPTER TEN

The AIDS Conspiracy

"At present the population of the world is increasing at about 58,000 per diem. War, so far, has had no very great effect on this increase, which continued throughout each of the world wars. . . War has hitherto been disappointing in this respect. . . but perhaps bacteriological war may prove effective. If a Black Death could spread through the world once in every generation, survivors could procreate freely without making the world too full. The state of affairs might be unpleasant, but what of it!"

— Bertrand Russell

By the summer of 1986 when I first met Strecker, the idea had already crept into the scientific literature that the AIDS epidemic might have been deliberately unleashed. Admittedly, one had to search hard to find published evidence for this accusation, but it was there if one pursued the leads.

I was fortunate to know Strecker because he frequently supplied me with obscure and mind-boggling AIDS reference material which greatly contributed to my understanding of a possible AIDS conspiracy.

After a busy day spent with patients, Strecker would often go the medical library at the University of

Southern California where he would spend many evenings combing the AIDS literature. There was very little of note that escaped his attention.

In 1985, a few scientists began openly to be critical of the government's handling of the epidemic. There were little rumblings of concern and discontent about the supposed origin of the AIDS virus and the source of the new epidemic. Only time would tell if these early insinuations of a government AIDS conspiracy and a scientific cover-up would quietly disappear, or eventually ignite a flame of public protest.

The first serious attack against the AIDS scientists came from America's arch enemy, Russia, in a commentary aired from a Moscow radio station on December 25, 1985. The highly inflammatory radio report, issued in English, concluded that "the AIDS epidemic has been caused by experiments carried out in the U.S.A. as part of the development of new biological weapons." The Russians cited the views of an English venereologist, John Seale, who was purportedly in agreement with the Soviet view of the laboratory origin of the AIDS virus.

In a "Letter to the Editor" published in the August 1986 issue of the *Journal of the Royal Society of Medicine*, Seale responded to the inflammatory Soviet claims. He readily admitted that the serious Soviet charges against the United States had forced him to clarify his own thoughts about the possibility that the AIDS virus could have been "man-made."

Seale made it clear that there was no real evidence to indict any specific scientific or military group. However, he did warn the scientific community to "reflect most carefully upon the Soviet statements."

Seale disagreed with Gallo's contention that the AIDS virus was a member of the HTLV (human T-cell leukemia/lymphoma virus) "family" of viruses. On the contrary, Seale was of the opinion that the AIDS virus was genetically closer to animal viruses (such as the "visna" virus of sheep) than it was to any "human" virus.

Theoretically, Seale had no doubt the AIDS virus could have been artificially created in a laboratory. In his view, an animal virus like visna could have been grown in cell tissue laboratory culture. Subsequently, the animal virus could have been transplanted into a human tissue cell culture. Scientists could then have injected this newly-created virus into *"humans used as guinea pigs."*

In 1978, scientists in virus laboratories had already performed experiments in which sheep visna virus was passed into human brain cells, thereby allowing the sheep visna virus to "jump" into a new species, *Homo sapiens.*

For years virologists had been taking human viruses and bioengineering them into animals. Seale claimed it would be simple to reverse the procedure, taking animal viruses and putting them into human beings.

SEALE WASN'T EXACTLY SURE WHERE THE AIDS VIRUS CAME FROM, OR WHO OR WHAT COUNTRY MIGHT HAVE RELEASED IT. BUT HIS THEORY WAS BASED ON THE FACT THAT "ANY DETERMINED PERSON, WITH ACCESS TO THE AIDS VIRUS IN ANY LABORATORY, COULD START AN EPIDEMIC IN ANY COUNTRY, WHICH THEREAFTER WOULD INEVITABLY SPREAD TO EVERY COUNTRY."

One month after publishing Seale's letter, the British Editors of the *Journal of the Royal Society of Medicine* published a letter from Strecker. He was honored that such a prestigious Society thought enough about his controversial ideas to allow publication of his views. It is unlikely that his unorthodox opinions would ever have been allowed to be published in American scientific journals.

In his letter Strecker questioned "the gospel" of the American AIDS experts who claimed the AIDS virus "arose spontaneously in monkeys." He asked facetiously whether the man-made "bovine-visna" virus should also be included in the same "family" as the AIDS virus. (Bovine-visna virus is a newly-created laboratory "recombinant" virus which was artificially manufactured by growing bovine leukemia virus together with sheep visna virus in tissue cultures of *human* cancerous leukemic bone marrow cells). STRECKER THEN SPECULATED THAT THE AIDS VIRUS MIGHT ACTUALLY BE "BOVINE-VISNA" VIRUS!

In strong words (for a scientific journal), Strecker single-handedly took on the AIDS establishment. "Where is the sorcerer to banish all the flood created by the apprentices of the World Health Organization, and the United States National Institutes of Health?" he asked.

I wondered how many readers of the *Journal* understood the accusatory implications of Strecker's remarks that were contained in his brief letter. If Strecker hadn't patiently explained to me, over and over again, his concept of how the AIDS virus could have been "made," I would have understood very little of his letter.

But some people must have understood very clearly the implications of Seale and Strecker's allusions because soon both physicians would attain notoriety, of a sort, in the London press.

On October 26, 1986, Seale's startling accusations appeared on the frontpage of the London *Sunday Express*. The headlines claimed — "AIDS MADE IN LAB SHOCK" — the world exclusive of the killer virus which escaped in a secret laboratory experiment.

The story caused a sensation. According to the *Express*, "the killer AIDS virus was artificially created by American scientists during laboratory experiments which went disastrously wrong — and a massive cover-up has kept the secret from the world until today."

Seale told reporters he was totally convinced "that the AIDS virus is man-made," and Strecker added that the virus "must have been genetically engineered."

Jacob Segal, an East Berlin microbiologist, was also interviewed for the story. Segal also insisted that the AIDS virus was man-made, and was probably spliced together by combining sheep visna virus with one of the newly-discovered human cancerous T-cell leukemia/lymphoma viruses. When asked about the widely-accepted green monkey theory of AIDS, the German professor quipped, "It's ludicrous and scientifically incredible — and has been promoted, I believe, by the U.S. government as part of the cover-up."

Until months later, very little was heard of the outrageous British accusations in the American media. However, *TIME* magazine did a little piece on the *Sunday Express* brouhaha, and interviewed Seale and Strecker about their "bizarre" views.

TIME (Infectious propaganda, November 17, 1986) cited Strecker's notion that the AIDS virus "originated in either a natural or an artificial combination of viruses." *TIME* wasn't specific on the details, but Strecker insisted (as always) that the visna virus of sheep was combined with the bovine leukemia virus of cattle to produce the "new" AIDS virus.

The cat was out of the bag but few people were taking the "propaganda" seriously. According to *TIME*, "AIDS experts scoffed at the far-fetched notion," and Washington "accused the Soviets of waging a disinformation campaign." With that, the case was closed.

The New Delhi *Times of India* picked up the *Express* story and turned it into an editorial published on November 17, 1986. The editorial was reprinted in its entirety in the *New York Native*, (January 19, 1987) for its readers.

The Indian editorial was harsh. "Recent reports of a controversy amongst biologists over the origin of the AIDS virus should make all those concerned about the grave danger of germ warfare sit up and take notice. . . the biologists contend that there is no known animal virus with all the features of the HTLV-I germ and that the AIDS organism is a combination of the parts of the genetic material of the Maedi-Visna virus of sheep, with parts of the bovine virus."

The New Delhi *Times* concluded: "The consequences of this are too horrifying to contemplate. These deadly germs represent, like nuclear weapons, agents of mass annihilation. The only thing to do with them is to ban them and get rid of them."

The *New York Native,* under the editorial supervision

of Charles Ortleb, had a reputation for publishing highly controversial views of AIDS that could never have been published elsewhere. In the August 25, 1986 issue, the *Native* published a disturbing article entitled "The AIDS view from Europe," by Jonathon Hallwag.

Hallwag was a rare breed of writer who believed "AIDS was simply too perfect to be true. . . with plot ingredients which fell too chillingly, and too neatly into place to be some casual 'accident' of nature." He bemoaned the killing-off of the gay community, and the discovery of a "substance" frequently found in gay blood which was "as vivid and unmistakable as the yellow star by which the Nazis identified the Jews." Hallwag reminded his readers that "nature never takes such perfect aim. But bullets do. And bullets are made by man."

Hallwag had just returned from Holland, and noted that most Dutch AIDS cases had been traced to sexual contact with Americans. The new and fatal "American disease" now made it difficult "for an American to find a willing Dutch sex partner, even with a gross of condoms in his hands."

To some Europeans, the AIDS epidemic was reminiscent of what they had experienced two generations ago during the reign of the Nazi Third Reich. Speaking for his European friends, Hallwag wrote: "Wake up your country. Tell them it can happen there. AIDS is just the opening volley. The Gays are the Jews of Europe, doomed to death to further the political ends of men every bit as cruel and ruthless and power-crazy as Hitler. Don't they see that?"

The idea of genocide against gay people has been a

familiar theme in the *New York Native*. An editorial by Charles Ortleb (February 23, 1987) reiterated this message. "We are in a holocaust. I believe that the government has orchestrated AIDS to achieve its religious and social goals. To my mind, people who think AIDS is an accident of nature are naive. They also consider me paranoid. I consider them to be fools of the same variety that pulled the wooden horse into the city of Troy."

By 1987 a few scientists like Matilde Krim publically theorized that a biological accident could have initiated the AIDS epidemic in gay men. In a published conversation with Larry Kramer (*Interview* magazine, February 1987), Krim speculated that AIDS could have originated from virus-contaminated batches of "gamma globulin" which were inoculated into gay men for the purpose of protecting them from hepatitis virus infection.

Krim is a well-known AIDS expert and cancer virologist associated with Sloan-Kettering Hospital in Manhattan. She is also co-chairperson of the American Foundation for AIDS Research (AmFAR).

In the interview, Krim tries to dispel the notion that gay men were the cause of AIDS in America. She explains that, "We probably gave it to gay men to start with, by inoculating them with infected gamma globulin, which is probably what happened." Krim postulates that gamma globulin in the early 1970s was made from "pooled" human blood brought in from Africa and the Caribbean.

At first, Krim (like Strecker) suspected that contaminated experimental hepatitis vaccine used in the New

York City trials in gay men might heve exposed them to the AIDS virus. But after "checking the dates" of the trials, she reasoned that "these trials started in '78 and '79." She dismissed the hepatitis connection because "that's too late; we already had cases then. The (AIDS) infection occurred at least five years prior to that. . . in the early 1970s."

Krim speculates, "The for-profit blood industry was buying blood from prisoners and from overseas, including Africa and the Caribbean." She reasons that the gamma globulin may not have been properly prepared and purified to kill the AIDS virus.

Kramer asked Krim why only gay men were initially infected with the AIDS virus. She replied, "No other group was so constantly, almost habitually, given gamma globulin, as gay men."

Krim maintains she is the only scientist who theorizes a gamma globulin connection to AIDS. She also claims she never heard scientists ask the question "Why gay men? Why?"

I admired Krim's courage for going out on a limb, but I found it hard to believe that she had never heard the question "why gay men" that every thinking homosexual in America has asked himself since the beginning of the "gay" plague.

The gamma globulin theory is food for thought, but it is unlikely that gay men were the exclusive recipients of gamma globulin, and equally improbable that only Manhattan gays would have received the "contaminated" batches. Furthermore, if African and Caribbean blacks, and prisoners harbored the AIDS virus in their blood that eventually made its way into commercial gamma globulin, why weren't any of *them* dying from AIDS in the early and mid-1970s?

THE FACT REMAINS THAT THE FIRST AIDS CASES IN AMERICA WERE DIAGNOSED IN GAYS IN MANHATTAN, A FEW MONTHS AFTER THE HEPATITIS B VACCINE TRIALS BEGAN IN MANHATTAN. If any of those men were directly injected and infected with the AIDS virus during the vaccine trials, they could have developed the disease quickly or could have sexually transmitted the virus to other gays. This could explain why AIDS started exclusively in New York City gays shortly after the experimental trials.

By early 1987, Krim was not the only expert to speculate that AIDS might be a biological "accident."

Penthouse magazine would seem to be an unlikely place to find a serious discussion of this possibility. However, Gary Null is a controversial and respected medical writer who often contributes serious and well-researched articles to the girly magazine. In a story entitled "Medical Genocide: The AIDS Panic," (*Penthouse,* April 1987), Null interviewed J. Anthony Morris, a leading virologist who had worked for the NIH and for the FDA in virus vaccine research.

According to Morris, "The AIDS virus has been around for years." He bases his statement "on the presence of the antibody in blood that was taken 40 to 50 years ago, and stored in an icebox."

Morris speculates on the connection between hepatitis B and AIDS by noting that "the AIDS virus began to appear around 1979, immediately following tests of the first hepatitis B vaccine."

Morris claims he wrote to CDC officials "to convince me that there is no causative connection between the introduction of the *experimental* vaccine into the homosexual population and the occurrence of AIDS in the same population." The CDC director purportedly wrote to Morris that, "He believed that there was no connection, but that the convincing evidence was just not available."

In short, Morris believes the *experimental* hepatitis vaccine (which was manufactured exclusively from infected gay "carriers" of the hepatitis virus) was contaminated with the AIDS virus.

Null thinks Morris' theory could be easily verified "by asking AIDS patients whether they ever received a hepatitis *experimental* vaccine. Instead, however, the government prefers to have us believe that sexual contact and intravenous drug use is responsible for the transmission of AIDS."

Although it is still rare to find scientists who believe AIDS is a biologic accident, it is not uncommon to find virologists who disagree with Gallo's classification of the AIDS virus. Aided by his friend, Max Essex of Harvard, Gallo was quick to classify his newly-discovered "AIDS virus" into a family of "human" viruses known as "human T-cell leukemia/lymphoma viruses" (HTLV).

BUT NOT ALL SCIENTISTS WERE CONVINCED THAT GALLO'S VIRUS WAS "NEW." AND NOT EVERYONE THOUGHT IT WAS "HUMAN." SOME SCIENTISTS WERE SUGGESTING (IF YOU READ BETWEEN THE LINES) THAT GALLO'S NEW HUMAN VIRUS HAD COME FROM "OLD," "ANIMAL" VIRUSES.

Although the AIDS virus was included in the same family as the human T-cell leukemia/lymphoma virus (HTLV-I), some Japanese scientists reported that the "human" leukemia virus behaved very much like the cattle virus — "bovine leukemia virus" (BLV). The Japanese claimed the bovine leukemia virus had a "close evolutionary relationship" to the human HTLV-1 virus. In addition, both viruses shared "several biological properties."

Another group of Belgian research scientists also discovered similarities between cattle BLV virus and the human leukemia/lymphoma viruses. In fact, the actual resemblance of both viruses was so "close," that the researchers suggested that the "animal" BLV virus should be classified and included in the new "human" family of HTLV viruses. To stress their conclusion, the Belgians titled their scientific paper "BOVINE LEUKEMIA VIRUS, A DISTINGUISHED MEMBER OF THE HUMAN T-LYMPHOTROPIC VIRUS FAMILY."

To me, it seemed clear that if you weren't a virologist you would never be able to determine the exact origin of all these "new" AIDS and cancer viruses. And it was quite apparent that the dividing line between "human" and "animal" viruses was nebulous, at best.

However, one thing was certain. The "human" AIDS virus was related to previously known animal cancer viruses. Exactly which animal it originated from depended on which virologist you chose to believe. Most American scientists meekly followed Gallo and Essex, and chose to believe AIDS came from green monkeys. But other equally reliable scientists preferred to think it originated from known cattle and sheep viruses.

Wherever "it" came from, I was reasonably certain it didn't "jump" into the human species. More than likely, it was "pushed" into *Homo sapiens* in some experimental virus laboratory, and then deliberately or accidentally got "out."

Strecker kept insisting the AIDS virus was a manufactured virus created in a cancer virus lab because part of the genetic structure and the "look" of the AIDS virus resembled bovine leukemia virus; other parts looked and acted like visna.

Although AIDS was an immunodeficiency disease, another part of AIDS resembled a nerve and brain disease. The immunodeficiency of AIDS was caused by the bovine leukemia part of the virus; the neurologic and "wasting" symptoms of AIDS came from the visna part of the AIDS virus.

It seemed the "science" of cancer virology was based on little more than a continuing series of lab experiments that created all kinds of new and deadly viruses. Virologists could play with their new and dangerous creations, much like children could play with "Dr. Cloner's Home Cloning Kit." In Strecker's mind, these genetic experiments of death would eventually destroy human life on the planet.

With AIDS, the impressive laboratory games have become a new scientific reality with worldwide implications. Scientists can now create all sorts of bioengineered viruses which can produce new diseases that people will be powerless to fight against.

With the proper technology you could plant these little seeds of genetic material into anything that was living, and you could devise "immunologic tests" to detect if the plantings were successful.

When enough time passed, no one could tell what viruses and what diseases were real, and what were artificial. And for those dying of these new viral diseases, it made little difference.

I began to notice the "word games" used to explain the virology and immunology of AIDS in "continuing medical education" articles designed to enlighten physicians about the "new" science of AIDS.

For instance, an AIDS "education" article designed for dermatologists contained the following informational details on the origin and classification of the AIDS virus:

"The AIDS virus seems to have arisen from a similar monkey virus. . .

(The virus) is also somewhat closely related to the lentivirus visna in sheep. . .

The virus is more distantly related to the human T-cell leukemia virus. . .

The virus is also more distantly related to other primate retroviruses isolated from wild and captive old world monkeys."

Strecker was right. It did sound like double-talk. If the AIDS virus is "closely related" to visna, why wasn't it classified with the sheep "family" of viruses? If the AIDS virus is "distantly related" to human viruses like HTLV-1, why was it put in a "human" family of viruses?

Where did the AIDS virus come from? The answer didn't depend on science, but on which scientist you wanted to believe.

Apparently I was not alone in my confusion. A

committee of viral taxonomists met in early 1985 to decide exactly which "family" of viruses the AIDS virus truly belonged to.

After a year of taxonomic struggle, the experts made their decision. The International Nomenclature Committee agreed that a new name be given to the causative agent of AIDS. No longer would the virus be known as human T-cell lymphotropic (or leukemia/lymphoma) virus (HTLV-3), or AIDS-related virus (ARV), or lymphadenopathy-associated virus (LAV). Nor would the new virus be given the simple name "AIDS virus." The Committee rejected that name because of "the fear surrounding the disease."

The thirteen-member committee could not agree on the specific "family" of viruses that the new AIDS virus belonged to. Nor was mention made of putting the new virus in the "monkey family" of viruses.

Despite the protestations of Gallo and Essex (the co-discoverers and namers of the original "HTLV-3" AIDS virus), the Committee decided to give the AIDS virus a brand new name and a new "family." From now on, the AIDS virus would be officially known as "the human immunodeficiency virus," or "HIV" for short.

The medical journals and AIDS experts quickly adopted the new term "HIV" for the AIDS virus. Within a few years, the AIDS virus already had more aliases than most criminals.

Strecker said all the name and family changes were meant to disguise the true origin of the deadly virus. Although the new name HIV officially classified the virus as "human," a big question still remained. Was the "human" AIDS virus born out of an "animal" virus in an animal retrovirus laboratory?

A decade after the cat experiments paved the way for the discovery of the "human leukemia and lymphoma viruses" and the AIDS virus, the CDC in its *AIDS Weekly* (February 10, 1986) commented on "AIDS in cats" and how cats could be a useful experimental model for AIDS. As they had done back in the 70s, the retrovirus researchers successfully injected AIDS virus into "virus-free" cats and allowed the virus selectively to attack T-cell populations. The virologists produced yet another new disease, this one called "feline acquired immune deficiency syndrome," or FAIDS for short.

As I mused over the recent production and discovery of cat (feline) AIDS, I thought of those "animal rights" people who march and carry signs outside of laboratories where animals are injured and killed for scientific purposes. I thought of my lovable cat who sleeps by my side, and who licks my face at dawn. And I found myself thinking maybe those "animal rights" people were not so crazy after all.

WHEN WERE THE KILLING EXPERIMENTS GOING TO TEACH US TO HEAL? WHY DO SCIENTISTS HAVE TO DESTROY SCIENTIFICALLY THE IMMUNE SYSTEM WHEN WE SHOULD BE LEARNING WAYS TO STRENGTHEN IT? It was all so insane!

We had literally studied the immune system to death, and none of our brilliant scientists had anything to offer to heal (or even improve) the immune systems of thousands of people who were dying of AIDS.

What were the scientists doing? With all their bizarre

theories on the origin of the AIDS virus certainly a "biologic accident" should have been added to their list. Had they all forgotten their 1973 "Biohazard" conference where they laid plans to monitor the future probability that a deadly cancer-causing laboratory virus would escape into the "general" population?

Was it an "accident" that the AIDS virus was "introduced" into American gays and into Haitians? Was it a lie that the AIDS virus "jumped species" into blacks in central Africa? Why did retrovirologists never mention a possible laboratory "accident" as the origin of the AIDS epidemic?

Was Strecker's "man-made" theory of AIDS any more ridiculous than the fanciful theory of AIDS transmission during Haitian voodoo sacrifical rites? Or any more unlikely than the theory that AIDS came to America because of bizarre and kinky and sinful sex practices — the same sex practices which had been going on since the dawn of civilization, but had never before started a biological holocaust?

Why would anyone or any group want to do such a thing? Any scientist would surely know that a virus deliberately "introduced" into gays would never "stay" in the gay community. Any scientific expert with the barest knowledge of human sexuality would understand that.

And there would be no cure for a "biologic accident" with one of the deadly viruses that were created in the cancer virus laboratories. The scientists knew that. THEY KNEW THEY COULDN'T STOP "IT" ONCE IT GOT OUT.

Strecker theorized these new bio-engineered viruses could be used by governments for population control, or for political control of large groups of people. The world of *1984* was already here, but we were too stupid to realize it.

There was no logic in the madness. NONE.

On April 19, 1987, the story appeared in my home-town paper, the *Los Angeles Times*. It was titled "Soviets sponsor spread of AIDS disinformation," and it was written by Kathleen Bailey, a deputy assistant secretary of state in the Washington Bureau of Intelligence and Research.

For the first time, many Californians read that the Russians were spreading an anti-American disinformation story claiming that the U.S. government had engineered the AIDS virus during biological warfare experiments. The public learned the biowarfare story had already made headlines in the London *Sunday Express* on October 26, 1986. As a result, the slanderous *Express* article was reprinted in major newspapers in over 50 countries, "promoting anti-Americanism."

Bailey never mentioned Strecker, but the opinions of John Seale were discredited by a Finnish AIDS expert, Jukka Suni, whose statement Bailey requoted from a Helsinki newspaper. "For years, I have read (Seale's) writings and I think he is imbalanced or rather crazy. He is a prophet of doom who has been getting worse year after year."

Bailey glosses over all the Soviet biowarfare claims with her declaration that, "For the educated public, the story still did not ring true. Most specialists in the field of viruses openly disputed the theory that the AIDS virus could technically have been produced in a laboratory — Soviet or American."

According to Bailey, many Africans believe that American scientists created the AIDS virus, and that they have been wronged. To quell the anti-American AIDS disinformation campaign, Bailey went to Africa.

Apparently she convinced one African official that the biowarfare story was untrue by "detailing for him the origin of the story and providing statements from leading scientists, including Soviets, on the impossibility of artificially creating the virus." Only then did the African change his view.

No American AIDS scientist was mentioned by name, but Bailey did interview one "prominent U.S. expert" who was frustrated in the matter. "My colleagues and I want to share our AIDS research findings with any nation in need. It is a bit difficult, however, to promote scientific exchanges with a government that is accusing you of having done something so vile as creating the virus."

In September 1987 Seale came to Los Angeles to express his views. Unfortunately, I did not hear him speak. A friend of mine who attended one of his presentations was shocked not only by his remarks but also by the printed handout material he presented to the audience.

Seale downplayed the idea that the AIDS virus was man-made, although he admitted it was technically feasible. He claimed he was frequently misquoted on this issue by the Soviets and by the media. Nevertheless, he admitted "the Soviets are correct when they state the AIDS virus could have been created in the laboratory as a lethal virus designed for mass slaughter of people."

However, Seale also stressed it was "equally likely that the AIDS virus evolved naturally."

I carefully studied Seale's "memoranda" that he presented to the London House of Commons (Problems associated with AIDS, Volume 3, minutes of evidence, 8 April - 13 May, 1987). In the document he declared that AIDS is "characteristically a blood transmitted infection which is only transmitted with difficulty during sexual intercourse." Furthermore, "the *illusion* that AIDS is essentially a sexually-transmitted disease arose from the first observations that AIDS appeared to affect only sodomites (i.e male homosexuals) with numerous partners." (Seale does not consider sodomy as true sexual intercourse). He claims that "male homosexual contact of the finger, penis, or tongue with the rectal wall of another man transmits the virus very easily."

Seale blames U.S. gays for introducing the AIDS virus into Britain by "infecting others by having frequent, efficient contacts — sodomy with strangers." He did not theorize how the AIDS virus was "introduced" into American gays, nor did he mention African AIDS in his memoranda.

Seale's homophobia reached unprecedented heights by his declaration that, "Homosexual men have been the most determined and effective in distorting the truth about AIDS". . . and that they form "*a type of secret society*" within the scientific and medical community. He further added, "Homosexual men have been the vectors of the virus throughout the western world and if it had not been for their activities very few people in prosperous countries would now be infected."

Seale suggested some "methods of control" to thwart

AIDS in Great Britian. "The most urgent step to be taken is to break the pervasive grip by homosexuals on the information and disinformation which has emanated for so long from the journals of science and medicine and from much of the media. Once this has been done, other scientists, doctors and politicians can stress accurately the reality of the situation. . . The only way to halt the spread of the virus is to identify all those who are infected *by compulsory testing.* Government must then take whatever steps are required to ensure that those infected do not pass the virus on to anyone else."

Undoubtedly, Seale will be remembered in AIDS history as the first physician of note to consider the possibility that the AIDS virus was man-made as a possible bioengineered biowarfare weapon. However, his complete avoidance of the important issues of African (heterosexual) AIDS transmission; his obvious fear and hatred of homosexuals; and his inability to account for the "origin" of the AIDS virus in gays, were serious flaws in the new kind of "AIDS science" he was proclaiming.

Although he was a venereologist, I could not comprehend his often-conflicting views on exactly how the AIDS virus was transmitted. He stressed that "AIDS is a contagious disease transmitted both *by direct physical contact* and indirectly by blood." And yet, he concludes that AIDS is *not* a sexually-transmitted disease. That didn't make any sense to me.

He seems to contradict himself when he writes: "The AIDS virus is transmitted with great efficiency by sexual contact which is focused in the lower intestinal tract. It can also be transmitted, but much less easily, by normal sexual intercourse, and even less easily *by person-to-person non-sexual contact.*"

Although I was completely disenchanted with some of Seale's pronouncements, Strecker was impressed with Seale's assessment of the AIDS problem. For the first time, Strecker and I were at odds in our thinking. Of course, he readily dismissed Seale's contention of a homosexual "secret society" and his belief that gays were spreading AIDS disinformation.

I suppose it was inevitable that we would have our first serious intellectual rift; it was impossible for two doctors to agree totally on anything. And AIDS was a volatile subject universally colored with personal prejudices and psychosexual conflicts.

Now that Seale had physically entered the picture, my ego was asking Strecker to choose sides. It was a dumb thing to do, and I soon realized what I was doing. Each of us was coming from a different place, and it was a call for tolerance and trust, not war.

Strecker had mixed feelings about the gay community and I tried hard to understand them. Privately, he chided the gays for not "waking up" to the real biowarfare origin of AIDS. He couldn't understand why gay political leaders and scientists never challenged the government's green monkey theory of AIDS. Why couldn't the gays understand that they were deliberately "set up" as both the victims and the perpetrators of the AIDS plague?

I also wondered why most gays were so unquestioning, but I imagined their situation was much like the Jews in Nazi Germany. The Jews thought if they cooperated with the Nazis, and did not challenge them they would be safe. Of course, they weren't.

American gays were relying on the government and the government scientists to save them. They wanted life, not death in government-sponsored concentration camps that they feared would be set up to stop the AIDS holocaust.

Could the AIDS epidemic be a clandestine war where biological agents of death were substituted for bullets and bombs? Was AIDS the inevitable outcome of a new consciousness on the planet that was scientifically creating socially acceptable methods for mass exterminations that would serve the economic and political needs of the world's most powerful governments?

Previous biowarfare experiments against civilians were already an historical reality. Military biowarfare attacks against unsuspecting civilians took place during the 50s and 60s in many parts of America. The most notorious was a six-day U.S. military bioattack on San Francisco in which clouds of potentially harmful bacteria were sprayed over the city. Twelve people developed pneumonia due to the infectious bacteria, and one elderly man died from the attack (Army germ fog blanketed S.F. for 6 days in '50 test, *Los Angeles Times*, September 17, 1979).

In other secret experiments, bacteria were sprayed in New York City subways, in a Washington, D.C. airport, and on highways in Pennsylvania. Biowarfare testing also took place in military bases in Virginia, in Key West (Florida), and off the coasts of southern California and Hawaii (Army used live bacteria in tests on U.S. civilians, *Los Angeles Times*, March 9, 1977).

It may be years before the public learns of similar experiments that have taken place in the 1970s, as part of the military's ongoing chemical and biological warfare program. In light of what is now known about previous biowarfare programs, the theory that AIDS is a covered-up biowarfare experiment should be given serious attention.

It should be obvious to biomedical investigators and researchers that finding the "truth" in biologic matters is becoming increasingly difficult, if not impossible, due to the fact that secret government-sponsored biological warfare experiments are now a commonplace reality.

In a letter to the editor of the *Journal of Epidemiology* (Volume 120, 1984, page 167-168), Irwin Bross bemoaned this state of affairs by calling attention to a new kind of "official" science that was taking the place of "genuine" science.

Bruss wrote: "In my view, the *Journal* has degenerated into little more than a house organ for 'official science'—for epidemiology that is supported by federal health and science agencies and produces 'findings' in line with the policies of those agencies. Like state religion, official science serves the interest of the state. Since the federal government is currently the adversary of its own citizens in litigation concerning the health effects due to misuse or abuse of radiologic, chemical, and medical tehnologies, this means that official science epidemiology serves the government interest, although this is against the public interest. SINCE 1955, OFFICIAL SCIENCE HAS BEEN STEADILY REPLACING GENUINE SCIENCE IN MANY AREAS, INCLUDING EPIDEMIOLOGY,

AND THE PROCESS BY WHICH TECHNICAL JOURNALS BECAME HOUSE ORGANS OF OFFICIAL SCIENCE WAS SO GRADUAL THAT FEW REALIZE WHAT HAS HAPPENED."

Philip Sartwell, an editor of the *Journal*, denied the charges by writing, "Perhaps Dr. Bruss had Orwell's *1984* in mind, and it is true that in a totalitarian regime such offenses would be possible, but they do not exist and have not existed in the *Journal*."

I had tried my best to make scientific sense out of the origin of the new AIDS holocaust. Despite my investigation, the exact origin of AIDS remained a mystery.

I had raised more questions than I had answered, and it was all deeply disturbing and depressing.

The planet was facing the most fearful epidemic since the great plagues of the Middle Ages, and nothing could be done to stop it.

It was ironic. Science — man's exalted substitute for God — had failed completely.

References:

Seale R: AIDS virus infection: A Soviet view of its origin. J Royal Soc Med 79:494-495, 1986.

Georgidis JA, Billiau A, Vanderschueren B: Infection of human cell cultures with bovine visna virus. J Gen Virol 38:375-81, 1978.

Strecker RB: AIDS virus infection. J Royal Soc Med

79, September 1986.

Sagata N, Ikawa Y: BLV and HTLV-I: Their unique genomic structures and evolutionary relationship, in Miwa M, et al (Eds), *Retroviruses in Human Lymphoma/Leukemia*, Japan Sci Soc Press, Tokyo/VNU Science Press, Utrecht, pp 229,240, 1985.

Burny A, Bruck C, Cleuter Y, et al: Bovine leukemia virus, a distinguished member of the human T lymphotropic virus family, in Miwa M, et al (Eds), *Retroviruses in Human Lymphoma/Leukemia*, Japan Sci Soc Press, Tokyo/VNU Science Press, Utrecht, pp 219-227, 1985.

Kaplan MH, Sadick N, McNutt NS, et al: Dermatologic findings and manifestations of acquired immunodeficiency syndrome. J Am Acad Dermatol 16:485-506, 1987.

CHAPTER ELEVEN

AIDS
and World Madness

As the number of AIDS deaths mounted to almost 25,000, and as the public hysteria intensified, I became convinced the AIDS epidemic was a good example of universal madness in one of its ugliest forms. AIDS had suddenly forced open the doors to everyone's sexual closet. Out poured the hatred, the fear, and the guilt that provided the scripts of our soap opera lives.

After years of study and research, I realized I was looking at AIDS with a curious mix of fascination and fear. AIDS was Pandora's box, and despite the danger, I wanted to open the lid and peer inside.

I had been seduced by the AIDS virus story. It was like the apple the serpent offered Eve. I wanted its power, knowing full well the virus contained the secrets of life — and the seeds of death.

Part of me hated the AIDS virus that had taken away so many of my friends. Some lingered on, valiantly fighting the disease for two years or more; others died quickly (and perhaps more mercifully) from Pneumocystis pneumonia. Although I occasionally heard rumors of people who were cured of AIDS, no one I knew with AIDS ever escaped death, no matter how hard they fought against the virus. The disease was always fatal.

Some men were in their sixties; others in their twenties and thirties. White, black, good-looking, homely, tall, short, masculine, effeminate, well-built or puny, educated or uneducated. It didn't matter. The virus was completely non-discriminating.

Within a decade the hot and hunky men who personified the fantasy sex symbols of the Gay Movement in America had toppled from their pedestals, and lay dead or dying. All the handsome youths, the hard bodies, the well-hung studs, the sexual supermen who had been the gods of sex and love had been transformed into idols of death; the so-called "body to die for." Only remnants of their former glory, immortalized on murky pornographic tapes, flickered on TV screens in lonely and darkened bedrooms.

Soon the sex goddesses and the macho gods of the straight world would also fall. The plague was the destroyer of all sex. From now on, sex and death would be blended into a new worldly reality, which would forever transform man's most powerful and most basic desire nature.

On Hollywood Boulevard I saw a young teenager wearing a T-shirt that symbolized the demise of sex in the late 1980s. As he walked past me, I shuddered as I read the message on his shirt.

$$\frac{\text{Love} + \text{Sex}}{= \text{AIDS}}$$

It seemed to say it all so simply and so tragically.

Now that the practice of medicine has become so intertwined with government politics, I sense a grave danger that medical science will become another weapon of destruction to be used against people who are deemed "biologically inferior."

At present, people with AIDS and persons who test "positive" for AIDS virus antibodies are in great peril from political forces who wish to remove these "infected" people from society. Such remedies and "solutions" recall to mind the reign of Nazi terror and the ensuing Holocaust. In order to purify the German "master race," millions of Jews, homosexuals, Gypsies, political dissenters, mentally retarded persons, and other "undesirables" were forced into concentration camps and exterminated for the good of the Third Reich. With the impending future horror of thousands of AIDS deaths, it would be easy to repeat the scenario of Nazi Germany once more on the planet.

As a physician, I am concerned about a new and dangerous kind of drug experimentation which encourages and justifies the use of AIDS patients as acceptable "treatment models" because AIDS is "invariably fatal." On TV, I watch Congressional Hearings on these new drug "protocols." I listen to the doctors, the scientists, and the pharmaceutical experts from the most powerful drug companies, and I strongly suspect that these "trials" in gay men are little more than a cruel hoax — a repeat of expensive and harmful anti-cancer drugs that did little, if anything, to heal cancer patients. And now these old toxic drugs are being resurrected in the hopes that they will somehow miraculously heal AIDS patients.

I read about experts who suggest celibacy as the only sure way to lessen the spread of the epidemic. And I listen to scientists who think that more money for research will stop AIDS. They talk like the same scientists who thought money would conquer cancer by 1976. And I see naive politicians on TV who think that a quarantine of two million Americans will stop AIDS, the same politicians who ignore the hundreds of thousands of homeless and mentally-disturbed people who roam the streets of our country.

And there are those who still believe in a forthcoming protective AIDS vaccine. But the experts acknowledge that a vaccine will be difficult, if not impossible, to make. Thus, the AIDS vaccine remains elusive, and will probably not be available until the next century, if at all.

I am angry about the madness I perceive in medical "science," the insanity of professional lives and careers devoted to the bioengineering of designer viruses of death.

I deplore the uncaring, unfeeling, and business-like attitude that is now so prevalent in the medical profession. As physicians, we have forgotten our Hippocratic oath to "Do No Harm," and we no longer remember that we are supposed to be healers. With our "controlled" scientific experiments, and our increasing disrespect for all forms of life, including our own, we have become doctors of death. We celebrate the never-ending experimental laboratory production of cancer and other deadly diseases. We incessantly document the countless deaths of laboratory animals we infect with our manufactured viruses.

Our high-tech laboratories of death attest to our

expertise as scientific destroyers of life. We blithely transfer infectious agents from species to species, and then we have the audacity to blame African green monkeys for the most deadly epidemic ever experienced on this planet.

We award our experimenters with the highest honors attainable in medical science, and we somehow expect their experiments of death to teach us to heal. How sad. How pathetic. How insane.

I am incensed about the virus that was mysteriously "introduced" into America — the so-called "monkey virus" which escaped from the steaming jungles of darkest Africa, and which mysteriously made its way to the island of Manhattan to target, attack, and destroy the immune systems of young gay men.

And in evaluating this new plague, I ask myself the scientific questions I was trained to ask in medical school.

Why were there no promiscuous heterosexuals among the early AIDS cases?

Now that we know women are also susceptible to AIDS virus infection, why were men the EXCLUSIVE victims of the new virus? And if intravenous drug abuse is "high-risk" for AIDS, why weren't drug addicts the FIRST people to get AIDS, instead of healthy, young gay men?

And most of all, I wonder why AIDS experts never ask themselves how a sexually-transmitted virus that spreads easily among heterosexuals could have started in America as an exclusively "gay" disease, transmitted only between male homosexuals.

HOW COULD TWENTIETH CENTURY, SOPHIS-

TICATED SCIENTISTS BELIEVE IN A VIRUS THAT SELECTIVELY TARGETS ONLY YOUNG GAY MEN? OR BELIEVE IN A GERM THAT HAS AN AFFINITY FOR HAITIANS? WHAT KIND OF A MICROBE "IN NATURE" PICKS ON WELL-DEFINED GROUPS OF PEOPLE? WHY CAN'T DOCTORS AND SCIENTISTS ADMIT THAT NO MICROBE "IN NATURE" ACTS LIKE THAT.

We are sitting on a biological time bomb. Strecker's prophecy that Africa is doomed is becoming a reality. The latest (1987) WHO estimates reveal that 50 to 100 million people worldwide are infected with the AIDS virus. Within five years, three million people will have AIDS. BY THE END OF THE CENTURY, IT IS PREDICTED THAT 50 MILLION AFRICANS WILL DIE FROM AIDS!

Each year, scientists predict that a higher and higher percentage of people who test positive for AIDS antibodies will die of the disease. In the beginning, it was estimated that 10% of "positive" people would die of AIDS; now the estimate is as high as 75%. Strecker believes that 100% of antibody carriers will eventually die of AIDS or AIDS related diseases. I hope he is wrong.

I am disillusioned with religious leaders and "good" people who argue that condoms and "safe sex" are against the laws of God, even though such measures may lessen the transmission of the AIDS virus. Why do church leaders insist that millions of people be allowed to risk death to keep from offending God? Have they somehow forgotten that all life is sacred to God who (if we are to believe the Bible) created it?

Along with the rest of the medical community, I am powerless to save the dying. It seems all we can offer is hope and compassion. But perhaps I am too pessimistic.

I recently learned a lesson about hope by talking with a man whose friend, Bill, had died of lung cancer some months earlier. The man told me how helpful I had been during the last weeks of Bill's life. He had been through radiation and chemotherapy, and the doctors told him there was nothing more they could do. Bill couldn't believe he was dying of lung cancer; he had never smoked a cigarette in his life.

Bill asked if I knew of anything he could do. Both of us knew his chances were one in a million, but I wanted to help him in some way. After mulling it over, I suggested he talk with Virginia Livingston. She was giving a lecture in Los Angeles, and I thought he might like to hear her views on cancer immunotherapy and her treatment program for cancer patients.

After the lecture, I introduced Bill to her. She was sorry to hear his diagnosis, but was willing to try and help him.

As the man talked about Bill's experiences at Virginia's clinic in San Diego, I interrupted and began to apologize for having suggested that Bill see Virginia so late in his disease.

But he stopped me. "No, you made Bill very happy. Dr. Livingston gave him some hope which he badly needed at the time. He followed her dietary advice, and he began to believe he had regained some control in fighting his disease. After he started on Virginia'a program he felt better about himself again. He was glad she tried to help him."

I was moved by the conversation. It reminded me how I had forgotten about "hope" and "faith" as therapy when all else had failed.

Later, as I thought more about it, I imagined that when one is near death there is only hope and faith: hope that one's life was not lived in vain; hope that something was accomplished; hope that something of ours might remain in the world that somebody could use; having faith that a spark of our identity lives on somewhere in the universe.

I have a physician friend, Barry, who can't stand to listen to all this AIDS conspiracy business. On his face are several tiny purple spots of Kaposi's sarcoma, the telltale sign of AIDS. I try to reassure him the cancerous spots could pass for pimples, at least for the present.

For a doctor, Barry has adopted a strange attitude about his disease: he simply denies it. Not completely of course, but as best as he can.

He refuses a skin biopsy. When I asked him why, he quickly answered, "Do you think I want my name on a Kaposi's sarcoma report sent to the government, so that some crazy politician or judge can lock me up, or quarantine me in some camp because they hate faggots with AIDS? No, thank you!"

Sometimes, he breaks down and cries like a baby, knowing that someday soon his purple spots will worsen, and that he will be shunned and treated like a leper.

Barry gets angry when I talk about Strecker's AIDS theories.

He argues, "How is all that conspiracy garbage going

to help me? This is MY disease. Knowing that someone might have given it to me deliberately doesn't help me one damn bit. In fact, I hate thinking about that crap. I only know I'm the only person who can take responsibility for my condition. No one's gonna do it for me. What you're telling me doesn't change a damn thing. It only makes it worse."

I have gotten into the habit of putting a cross next to the names of friends in my address book who have died of AIDS. I keep telling myself I need to buy a new address book, but then their names would be gone forever.

Perhaps it's morbid, but the crosses help to keep them alive in my mind. Under "A" is one cross. "B" has three, "C" and "D" each have two crosses. The crosses remind me how lucky I am to be alive.

The experts say that if you are in a "high risk" group you should be tested to find out if you have been exposed to the AIDS virus. But they don't tell you that you have a 50:50 chance of dying of AIDS if you're positive. Or how to keep a positive attitude about life when you have a virus in your body that is designed to destroy your immune system.

We have done a great job of screwing up the planet. We've messed up the earth, the waters of the rivers and oceans, the air we breathe (and even the ozone layer), the food we eat, and now we've messed up love. Is there any doubt the planet needs healing?

I have thought deeply about my motives for writing

this book. Did I write it out of love, or out of hate? Perhaps it was out of a love for truth and a hatred of deception.

I only know the book had to be written. In some ways, it was a personal catharsis; a partial release from all the anger and frustration I feel about the many senseless deaths from AIDS.

Some friends said I shouldn't write this book because it might anger people. It could be dangerous.

As a scientist, I naively asked myself why questioning the origin of AIDS might make some people angry.

Who was really to blame for starting AIDS? Was it African green monkeys as they all said? Or did the germ-warfare scientists start it? Or the military biological warfare experts, or the CIA? Or maybe the Russians? Aren't the Soviets always to blame for America's international woes?

Where was the absolute proof for Strecker's theory that AIDS was a biological warfare experiment?

Was there a cover-up? Theoretically, AIDS could have been initiated by a few people in positions of power and influence. It would be easy to devise a simple biologic "accident" with contaminated vaccines.

Wouldn't the ones who created the mistake also create the cover-up? In the summer of 1987 the Iran-Contra Congressional Hearings proved to the public how dishonest and disloyal high-ranking government officials could be, and how diabolic and treasonous acts could be efficiently "covered up" by "good" people.

With the ever-increasing severity of the epidemic, I noticed more and more people withdrawing from each other. At times, I felt a loneliness that I had never experienced so acutely.

Paradoxically, in my feeling of isolation, I became more deeply aware of the connectedness of all peoples on this planet. Over and over, I was reminded that we were all facing this terrible epidemic together, whether we like it or not.

With the omnipresent AIDS virus, our sex lives, which once symbolized earthly pleasure and happiness, are now tainted with the specter of death.

With AIDS, I see a world of suffering now that so many young people are dying. And I seek desperately to understand the roots of the holocaust, and the way to outwit it.

I think of my life before this horrible epidemic, and it reminds me how lucky I have been because so many kind people have loved me. Without them, life would have been very painful.

Perhaps the mystics are correct. Perhaps the only reason we are here is to extend love. Because without love, the history of the human race has taught us it is easy to murder and destroy.

But what about people who never seem to find love?

Experts in psychology say that people with AIDS often feel unloved. Psychics tell us that many persons with AIDS are disenchanted with their worldly experiences. Lacking love, they want to move onto something else more satisfying.

I wonder if more people with AIDS would be encouraged to live if we offered them more in the way of love. But with all the current fear and hate, it is hard to give them the love they need.

One thing I'm sure of. If we loved ourselves more, we could love others better.

I wish I knew the true meaning of human sexuality. The more people you ask about sex the more confusing it gets. No one seems to know for sure. Perhaps each of us is supposed to seek and find our own truths about sex and loving.

I'm sure most people would agree that sex is part of love, but it's obviously not the same as love because it's normal to love people without being sexual with them.

We spend so much time and energy arguing about sex and love. And it seems ironic that our church leaders who claim to be asexual, celibate, or monogamous, regard themselves as supreme authorities on sex and love. Each religious leader claims his truths are the only correct ones, and all of them supposedly speak for God.

I have found it impossible to discover the true meaning of love and sex by asking others. Faithful and monogamous persons often claim their way of loving is best. Promiscuous people claim that loving more than one person can be a better experience. And some celibates insist that no sex is the ultimate physical and spiritual goal.

There are books expounding the joys of heterosexuality, homosexuality, bisexuality, and asexuality. And there are gays who think they are better than straights, and vice versa. And bisexuals who claim to have the best of both worlds.

Although many religious leaders attempt to judge love, there is little agreement among them. Therefore, it seems impossible to judge love, especially when we are unable to agree on what love is. Christian teachings suggest we should love one another, and not judge. That seems reasonable.

The rapid spread of AIDS throughout the world proves how connected we are to one another, if only by bodies. If only love could spread among us as easily and as quickly as the AIDS virus, the world would be a fabulous place.

What do we really know about AIDS? The fact that scientists originally believed (and convinced the public) that AIDS had an intrinsic connection to male homosexuality indicates that the AIDS experts did not understand the true nature of the disease. We now know that AIDS has nothing to do with homosexuality. It has only to do with acquiring the virus from an infected person.

It is becoming increasingly clear that there are additional facts about AIDS that the experts failed to understand.

They said it is a disease of "high risk" groups. The fact is AIDS is a disease that can affect anyone.

They said it posed little threat to the "general public." That is totally false. AIDS is now the leading cause of death in young men and women in New York City.

They said it is due to anal sex, drugs, and semen. It's not. It's due to a virus.

They said it is a disease of promiscuity. That's not always true. A monogamous person can get AIDS from an infected partner.

They said it was a hard disease to catch. By 1988, over 40,000 Americans had caught the disease, and millions more were infected.

Ignoring the experience in Africa and Haiti, some AIDS experts still say an infected woman can't give AIDS to a man.

The experts said there would be a vaccine available in 1986. No vaccine is expected until the next century.

They said the disease wasn't cancer, and that cancer was never "catching." But AIDS is "catching." And AIDS can lead to Kaposi's sarcoma, and Kaposi's sarcoma is cancer.

Finally, the general public is getting the message that everyone is at risk for AIDS. The only exceptions are couples who have been mutually monogamous since 1978 (the year the hepatitis vaccine trials began in gay men in New York City).

Now that AIDS has spread quickly to "straight" America, it has become the most fearful disease of our time. Artificial and imaginary boundaries no longer separate the "gay" and the "straight" world. People of all sexual persuasions have literally come together to produce an epidemic which will forever change our sexual attitudes, and further blur our neat little misconceptions of heterosexuality, homosexuality, and bisexuality. In short, we have met the enemy and it is us.

The tragedy of the AIDS epidemic is just beginning. How each of us deals with the disease in the coming years will determine its outcome.

There are many religious people who sincerely believe that AIDS is God's judgment and punishment against gays, drug addicts, prostitutes, immoral people, and other undesirables. Physicians have publicly joined in the condemnation of gays and other unfortunates with AIDS.

A Georgia physician, quoted in *MD* magazine (January 1987), says, "AIDS represents the consequences of violating God's rules regarding sexuality."

A Pennsylvania surgeon writes, "We used to hate faggots on an emotional basis. Now we have a good reason."

An internist from Oklahoma insists, "Homosexuality is a sin, deserving the death penalty."

The hatred and judgmental attitudes of those who claim to speak for God seem unalterable.

I never felt comfortable with the concept of a hateful, angry, and vengeful God. Although I was taught as a child to believe in such a God, I now prefer to think of God as Someone or as some Divine force who loves us all equally, totally, and eternally.

If GOD IS LOVE, and if we are part of Him, and if He is part of us, then perhaps the antidote to AIDS can be found in extending our love to one another.

It seems to me we have two choices. We can choose to be healers, and doctors of life. Or we can continue the epidemic as we began it — as practitioners of hate, punishment, guilt, and sin. And as unforgiving doctors of death.

We can choose the madness of sickness and death — or the joy of life and love.

The health of the planet depends on our collective decision.

Epilogue

In October 1987, a remarkable book entitled *And The Band Played On; Politics, People and the AIDS Epidemic* was published. The author Randy Shilts, a gay man and the first reporter to cover the AIDS story full-time, has written an exquisitely detailed historical account of AIDS which should be read by all serious students of the epidemic.

Much of what Shilts has to say is profoundly disturbing: the unwillingness of the scientific and medical community to take the new "gay plague" seriously, the political infighting between the various federal health agencies, and the shameful refusal of the Reagan administration to fund AIDS research and education, all combine to provide a serious indictment against the government's handling of the AIDS holocaust. Even more frightening is that these conditions remain essentially unchanged.

In the AIDS crisis of the late 1980s, the gay community is experiencing a catch-22 of the most perplexing sort. On one hand, gays seek to preserve the sexual freedom and political gains that were hard-won in the battle for gay rights during the 1970s. On the other hand, gays are faced with losing all these gains because of a sexually-transmitted virus that is decimating their numbers.

Despite all this, the gay community does not escape Shilts's subdued anger. He chronicles the petty political infighting among homosexuals, particularly around the volatile issue of closure of the gay bathhouses as a means to halt the spread of the deadly AIDS virus.

And The Band Played On has been widely praised as a remarkable work of journalism. Unfortunately, the book is likely to be best remembered for promoting the story of "Patient Zero"—a promiscuous, young gay Canadian airline steward named Gaetan Dugas—who is theorized as the man who brought the AIDS virus to North America. Already Shilts's Patient Zero theory has become another instant media AIDS "fact."

Despite the unbelievable collective imcompetence of public health officials which Shilts describes, he nevertheless relies on dubious anecdotes supplied by CDC epidemiologists and New York physicians which purport to link Dugas to the first reported AIDS cases. In this regard, the matter of Patient Zero is a serious flaw in Shilts's otherwise excellent tome.

The epidemiological finding of homosexual "links" between Dugas and some early cases of AIDS is not surprising in view of the fact that the AIDS virus is easily transmitted sexually. However, one should not infer from this data that Dugas "brought" AIDS to America.

Although Shilts admits his Patient Zero theory remains "a question of debate and ... ultimately unanswerable," he still claims Dugas brought AIDS from Paris to North America and "no doubt ... played a key role in spreading the new virus from one end of the United States to the other."

Medical reports found outside Shilts's book suggest otherwise. AIDS experts generally agree the AIDS virus originated in central Africa and was first "introduced" *exclusively* into the gay male population of Manhattan, somewhere around 1978-1979. Now (with no evidence) Shilts is proposing a brand new theory that Dugas "acquired" the virus in Paris and brought AIDS to America. Gaetan Dugas was diagnosed with Kaposi's sarcoma (i.e. AIDS) in June 1980 in New York City. He had swollen lymph nodes and a "rash" for one year before his diagnosis. Unmentioned by Shilts are medical reports that indicate the AIDS virus was already "in" the New York City gay community, two years before Dugas was diagnosed.

As evidence for this, we now know that Cladd Stevens and her group from the New York City Blood Center have traced the first and earliest known "positive" AIDS virus antibody tests back to young Manhattan gays who were injected with the hepatitis experimental vaccine at the Blood Center beginning in November 1978. Reexamined blood specimens taken during 1978-1979 show "positive" AIDS virus antibodies in 6.6% of those men injected with the experimental hepatitis vaccine (*JAMA*, Volume 255, pp 2167-2172, 1986). *In 1980, the year Dugas was diagnosed with AIDS, twenty percent of the Manhattan men in the experimental hepatitis vaccine study were "positive" for AIDS virus antibodies!* There is no conceivable way Dugas could ever have infected such a large number of New York City gays, as early as 1978-1979.

As expected, the media, apparently unconcerned with these aspects of AIDS science, sensationalized the story and "facts" of Patient Zero. *TIME* (October 19, 1987) reviewed Shilts's book in its "medicine" section as "The Appalling Saga of Patient Zero." The cover illustration of *California* magazine showed a shadowy airline steward, suitcase in hand, descending from a plane ramp as "Patient

Zero: The Man Who Brought AIDS To California." The bold headlines of the *New York Post* (October 6) read: "THE MAN WHO GAVE US AIDS—triggered gay cancer epidemic in U.S." Not to be outdone, The *Star* featured Dugas as "The Monster Who Gave Us AIDS," and referred to him as "a modern typhoid Mary—the man who infected a continent with AIDS." Even the AMA *American Medical News* (October 23) fell for the story, claiming that Dugas "may have brought AIDS to the United States."

Despite the overall brilliance of *And the Band Played On*, Shilts's account of patient zero seriously undermines the worth of the book, and serves as an example of how AIDS "facts" can be twisted and distorted to suit various political, social, moral, and even literary purposes.

During the first decade of the epidemic, we have been subjected to the highly dubious "African green monkey" theory of the origin of AIDS. What we don't need is any more AIDS myths in the guise of Gaetan Dugas—"the man who brought AIDS to North America."

What we do desperately need is a credible scientific explanation of how young, predominantly white, previously healthy homosexual men in Manhattan could have been the EXCLUSIVE RECIPIENTS of an AIDS virus that purportedly arose in black heterosexuals in central Africa.

To blame the origin and spread of American AIDS on one promiscuous airline steward (out of the thousands of heterosexual, bisexual, and homosexual airline stewards who fly around the world) seriously strains Shilts's credibility. It is this lapse of reason that keeps *And the Band Played On* from being the great book it could have been.

While the media had a field day with the Dugas gay scandal, a few short articles were printed concerning speculations that cattle AIDS-like viruses might be connected to the epidemic of AIDS. Scientists could no longer ignore the possibility that human vaccines might be contaminated with cattle viruses because such vaccines were produced, in part, from the blood serum of fetal calves.

According to Peter Drotman, a CDC epidemiologist, "There are some zealots who have made the suggestion that animal viruses are related to AIDS. None of these have been supported by any scientific evidence." (*New York Times*, October 22, 1987).

The *Times* briefly mentioned the 18 year-old cattle virus that was suspect. The cow virus had a brand new name that was reminiscent of the newly-named AIDS "HIV" (human immunodeficiency virus)—it was called bovine immunodeficiency virus or "BIV," for short. Scientists at a company in Frederick, Maryland (the site of the Army biowarfare program) would be conducting studies on BIV "under contract to the National Institutes of Health."

Newsweek (Bad Vaccines?, November 2, 1987) ran a tiny blurb on the subject of BIV contamination and the fact that it was "closely related to the human AIDS virus." A question was posed: "Could any of the world's stock of vaccines be contaminated by animal retroviruses similar to AIDS?" No mention was made of previous charges that smallpox vaccinations might have triggered AIDS in Africa, but the magazine mentioned that Jeremy Rifkin and his Foundation on Economic Trends were petitioning the World Health Organization to test its smallpox vaccines for such contamination. Rifkin "is especially concerned about vaccines cultured in cows."

I asked Strecker about "BIV." No listing appeared for

the 18 year-old cattle virus in my retrovirus textbook, published in 1985 by the Cold Spring Harbor Laboratory. Strecker thought the virus they were referring to was bovine-visna—a virus of obscure origin. He added it would be hard for me to find anything about BIV in the scientific literature.

It was a familiar story by now. All these strange old and new viruses popping up with new names and peculiar pedigrees and origins that no one was anxious to discuss.

At the end of 1987, 45,000 people had been diagnosed with AIDS. Twenty-five thousand had died of a disease that was supposedly "hard to catch." Almost 30% of the cases were from New York City, the site of the first (1978) hepatitis B vaccine trial.

Eight years after the first case was diagnosed in Manhattan, it was discovered that *AIDS had killed more intravenous drug addicts than homosexuals in the city.* For some reason, 2,520 drug-related AIDS cases had been left out of the "official" statistics. The New York City Health Commissioner was "absolutely startled."

With the *revised* statistics, IV drug abusers currently comprise 53% of the total 12,000 New York City cases; homosexual and bisexual men comprise 38%.

Now that IV drug abusers were discovered to be more "at risk" than non-drug using gay men, I wondered if epidemiologists would ask themselves why no IV drug abusers were among the earliest reported AIDS cases.

The AIDS virus slowly continues to reveal its deadly nature. Insurance companies are in the business of precisely predicting the longevity of their customers. The companies are determined to weed out applicants infected with the

228

AIDS virus. Their reasoning is not hard to understand. A 1987 insurance industry study showed that *a 35 year-old man with AIDS virus antibodies was fifty-one times more likely to die prematurely than an otherwise healthy man of the same age.*

Alice would have found the AIDS stories "curiouser and curiouser." There was really no way to understand fully the AIDS "science" and pseudoscience that pervaded the medical journals and the popular magazines.

There is only one way to make sense of the insanity surrounding the AIDS epidemic ... and that is to realize that we are at war with one another. And it is well to remember that the "truth" in wartime is often neatly packaged to delude the masses.

With the AIDS war there are no bombs, no bullets, and no visible signs of destruction. But the number of mass deaths are climbing steadily as predicted and as planned.

The "high risk" people are slowly disappearing. It is possible they will all be put away eventually in camps by authorities who are advocating new laws requiring quarantine of those infected with the virus.

"High risk" is a propaganda word used to mark and to mask the genocide of well-defined groups of people who are not well-liked in America. It is a replay of the deaths of millions of "undesirables" who quietly vanished in Europe under the yoke of Nazism—and no one outside of Germany ever knew about their plight until years later when it was too late.

The AIDS story was more diabolic than any Hollywood script writer could ever devise. People like Strecker and me who intuitively recognized the insanity of the epidemic

229

would be ignored as crazy paranoid individuals—and would be shunned along with the sick and infected.

It was a silent war unlike any war ever experienced by mankind. *It had all the characteristics of biological warfare.*

It was ironic. We were all in it, and yet it didn't seem like a war. It seemed more like an illusion ...

Perhaps with more time, the meaning would be clear to everyone. Or perhaps the madness would always continue, as it always has on this planet, until we wake up to the Truth.

INSTITUTIONAL
ABBREVIATIONS

American Cancer Society   **ACS**
American Medical Association   **AMA**
American Psychiatric Association   **APA**
Centers for Disease Control, Atlanta   **CDC**
Central Intelligence Agency   **CIA**
Federal Bureau of Investigation   **FBI**
Federal Drug Administration   **FDA**
International Agency for
Research on Cancer   **IARC**
National Cancer Institute   **NCI**
National Institute for Allergy and
Infectious Diseases   **NIAID**
National Institutes of Health   **NIH**
United States Public Health Service   **USPHS**
World Health Organization   **WHO**

Subject Index

Index of Proper Names

236

237

Pape, Jean 133
Pasteur Institute 58-60
Paxman, Jeremy 70
Pennsylvania 203
Penthouse magazine 190
People magazine 161
Philippines 163
Pope John Paul II 103, 144
Proceedings in Clinical and Biological Research 102

R
Rapoza, Norbert 118-125
Rappoport, Jon 134
Rauscher, Frank 32-33, 42
Reagan, Ronald 171, 223
Reich, Wilhelm 7
Rife, Royal 7
Rifkin, Jeremy 227
Rivers, Eunice 170
RNA Tumor Viruses 181
Russell, Bertrand 175
Russia (see Soviet Union)
Russian Academy of Medical
  Science 105

S
St. John, Ronald 133
St. Louis 99
St. Louis Sexually-Transmitted
  Disease Center 77-78
San Francisco 17, 44, 67-69, 84,
  91, 94, 97, 99, 106, 119, 131, 203
San Francisco City Clinic 77-78
Sartwell, Phillip 205
Science magazine 59, 148, 150,
  174
Scientific American 111
Seale, John 182-183, 185, 198-202,
  216
Segal. Jacob 185
Seibert, Florence 7
Shilts, Randy 223-226
Shogun 178
Sloane-Kettering Hospital 188
Slot, Larry 150
Soviet Union 74, 101-105, 182,
  198-200, 216

Stanley, James B 72
Star, The 226
Stevens, Cladd 89-90, 92-95, 225
Strecker, Robert 20, 22-30, 36-
  37, 45-46, 69-70, 73, 84-85, 97-
  99, 106, 111-112, 134-135, 150-
  152, 171, 176, 179, 181, 184-186,
  188, 193-195, 197-198, 202, 212,
  227-229
Strecker, Ted 24-25
Sunday Express (London) 185,
  198
Suni, Jukka 198
Szmuness, Wolf 74-75, 89, 101-105

T
Teas, Jane 126
TIME magazine 57, 111, 185-186
Times of India (New Delhi) 186

U
U.S. Army Department of Biological Warfare 71, 227
U.S. Department of Agriculture
  176
U.S. Public Health Service 31, 86, 168

V
Vieira, Jeffrey 128
Vietnam 165
Virginia 204

W
Washington, D.C. 88, 100, 120, 203
Washington Times, The 150
Weiss, RA 118
West Germany 164
Wheeler, Owen 23
White, Dan 68-69
WHO (see World Health Organization)
World Health Organization
  (WHO) 67, 71, 104, 113-115, 122,
  133-134, 138, 184, 227

Y
Yale University School of Public
  Health 41, 104

Z
Zaire 125
Zambia 117

About the Author

Alan Cantwell is a dermatologist and scientific researcher in the field of cancer and AIDS microbiology. He is a graduate of New York Medical College, and studied dermatology at the Long Beach Veterans Administration Hospital in Long Beach, California. Doctor Cantwell is the author of more than thirty published papers on cancer, AIDS, and other immunological diseases, which have appeared in leading national and international, peer-reviewed medical journals. His writings have appeared in *Organica, Paranoia, Steamshovel Press,* and the *New African.* He is also the author of *AIDS: The Mystery and the Solution* (1984), *The Cancer Microbe* (1990), *AIDS & The Doctors of Death* (1988), and *Queer Blood* (1993), all published by Aries Rising Press. Japanese language editions of *AIDS and the Doctors of Death* and *Queer Blood* have recently been published in Tokyo. Doctor Cantwell was born in New York City in 1934, and now lives in Los Angeles.